THE PHALLUS

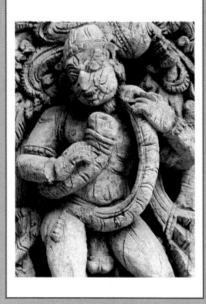

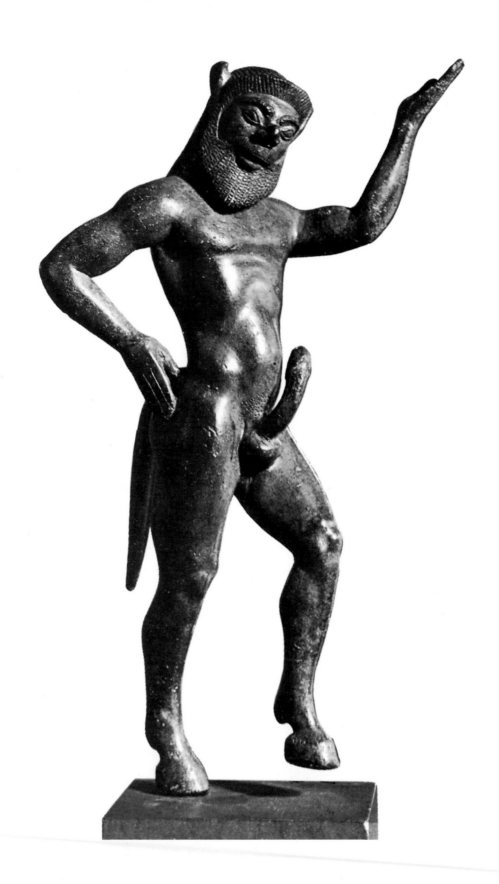

THE PHALLUS

◆

SACRED SYMBOL OF
MALE CREATIVE POWER

◆

ALAIN DANIÉLOU

TRANSLATED BY JON GRAHAM

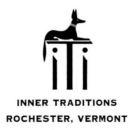

INNER TRADITIONS

ROCHESTER, VERMONT

INNER TRADITIONS INTERNATIONAL

ONE PARK STREET
ROCHESTER, VERMONT 05767

Originally published in French by Pardes, Puiseaux, France,
in 1993 as *Le Phallus*
Translation copyright © 1995 Inner Traditions International

LIBRARY OF CONGRESS CATALOGING-IN-PUBLICATION DATA
Daniélou, Alain.
[Phallus. English]
The phallus : sacred symbol of male creative power / Alain Daniélou ;
translated from the French by Jon Graham.
p. cm.
Includes bibliographical references.
ISBN 0-89281-556-6
1. Penis—Religious aspects. 2. Phallicism. I. Title.
BL460.D3613 1995
291.2'12—dc20   95-22029
                                                           CIP

Printed and bound in Canada

10 9 8 7 6 5 4 3 2 1

Text design and layout by Bonnie F. Atwater

This book was typeset in Berling Agency with OPTIProtea,
Copperplate, and Bernase as display fonts.

Distributed to the book trade in Canada by Publishers Group West (PGW), Toronto, Ontario
Distributed to the book trade in the United Kingdom by Deep Books, London
Distributed to the book trade in South Africa by Alternative Books, Randburg
Distributed to the book trade in Australia by Millennium Books, Newtown, N.S.W.
Distributed to the book trade in New Zealand by Tandem Press, Auckland

page i: India: Shiva as youth with elongated phallus. Photograph by Lance Dane.
page ii: Italy: Etruscan ithyphallic satyr. Bronze. National Museum, Athens.
pages 2 and 3: Corsica: Standing stones in phallic form. 3000 B.C. Photograph by Louis Trémellat.
pages 44 and 45: Jutland: Cernunnos, lord of the animals. Detail of the Gunderstrup cauldron, 100 B.C.
National Museum of Copenhagen.
Chapter opening ornament images of phallic sheaths photographed by Lance Dane.

In all cases the publisher has made every effort to contact and get permissiom from the artists and
appropriate institutions for the images and photographs in this book. Nevertheless, if omissions or
errors have occurred, we encourage you to contact Inner Traditions International.

CONTENTS

PART 2

◆

THE ITHYPHALLIC GOD

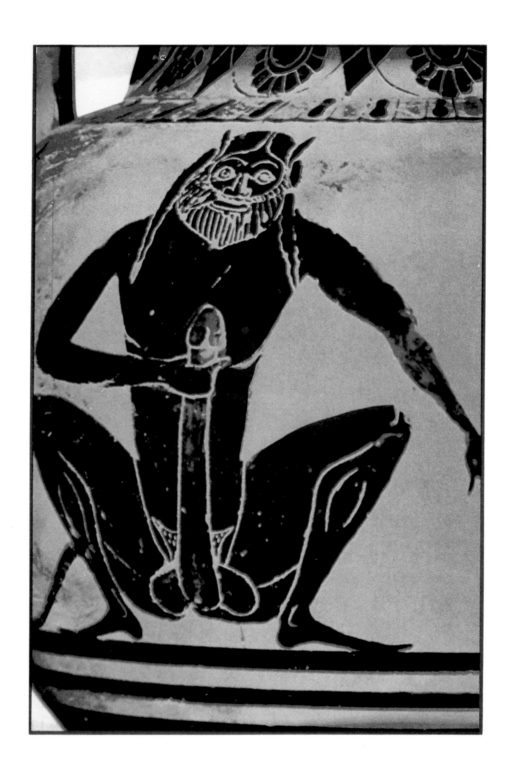

INTRODUCTION

It is only when the penis *(upastha)* stands up straight that it emits semen, the source of life. It is then called the phallus *(lingam)* and has been considered, since earliest prehistory, the image of the creative principle, a symbol of the process by which the Supreme Being procreates the Universe.

This is not a case of a symbol plucked at random but the recognition of the continuity of the process that links all the various levels of manifestation, according to cosmological theory. The phallus is really the image of the creator in mankind, and we rediscover the worship of it at the origin of every religion.

A source of pleasure, the phallus evokes divine bliss, the Being of Joy. Within the microcosm of the living being it represents the progenitor, which is always present in its work.

Contempt for this sacred emblem, as well as degradation and debasement of it, pushes man from the divine reality. It provokes the anger of the gods and leads to the decline of the species. The man who scorns the very symbol of the life principle abandons his kind to the powers of death.

◆

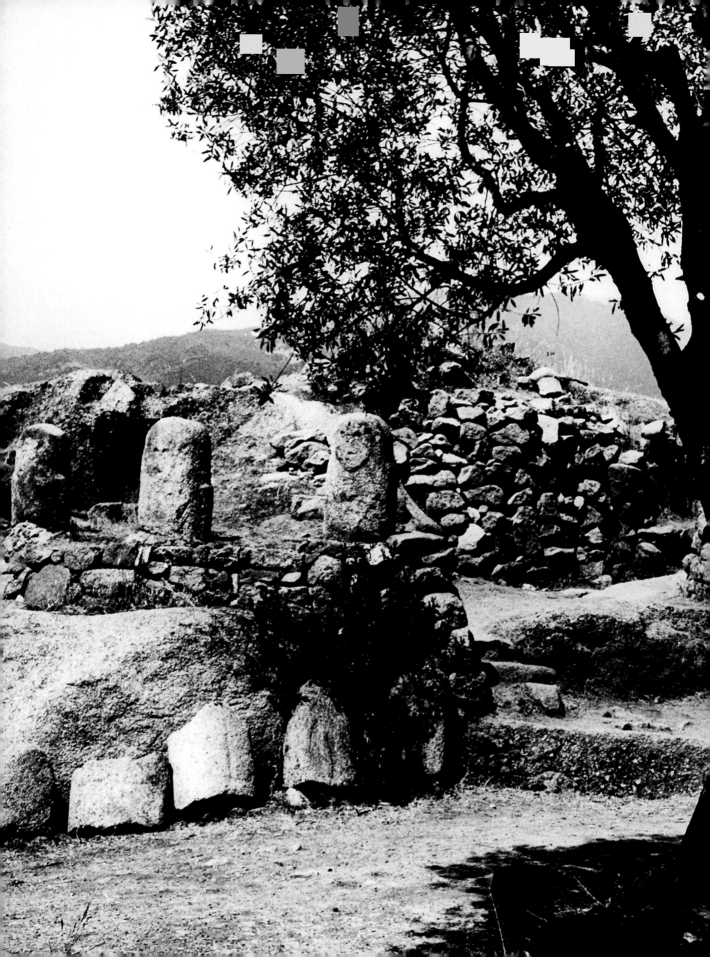

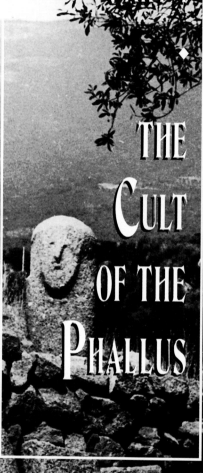

PART 1

THE Cult OF THE Phallus

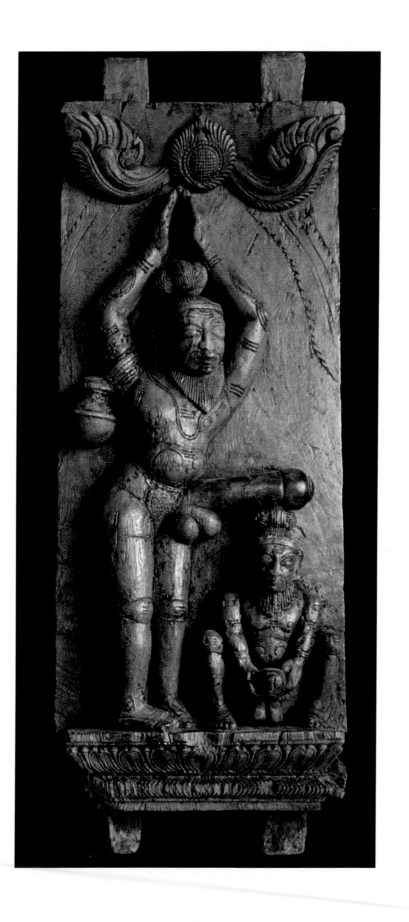

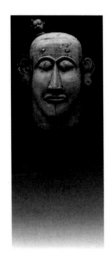

1

◆

HISTORICAL SOURCES

The cult of the phallus, the source of life and a symbol of virility, courage, and power, first appeared in the vast civilization that developed from India to the extreme edge of western Europe at the beginning of the Neolithic era following the end of the Ice Age about 8000 B.C. Closely tied to the bull and serpent cults, it has survived in India, with its rites and legends intact, to the present time, but its traces, symbols, and certain other cult elements can be discerned throughout not only all the civilizations of Mesopotamia, the Middle East, Egypt, and the Aegean but also those of Thrace, Italy, and the entire pre-Celtic world, including Ireland.

It is difficult to determine whether even more ancient sources existed in the immense history of humanity before the coming of our ancestor Cro-Magnon Man, which is to say before the debut of our own civilization, which thoroughly remains under its influence. The red horns that Italian drivers attach to the fronts of their trucks to avert misfortune, even today, are analogous to those used more than six thousand years ago by chariot drivers.

Among the cave paintings and carvings of the Paleolithic era, ritual representations of the feminine principle are especially noticeable. The

OPPOSITE
India: Youth with elongated phallus. Photograph by Lance Dane.

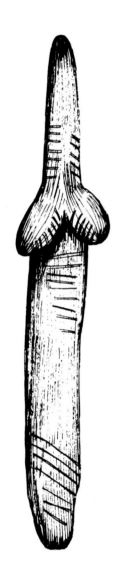

Moravia: Phallic amulet of Dolni Vestonice. Gravettian culture, 30,000 B.C.

man with the head of a bird and erect phallus of Lascaux (circa 20,000 B.C.) seems to be the exception. From the beginning of the Neolithic era, on the other hand, there are countless representations of the phallus and of ithyphallic figures, such as those of Altamira, Gourdan, and Isturits.

Jacques Dupuis has suggested in his latest book, *Au Nom du Père*, that this passage from worship of the vulva to that of the phallus could be linked to the discovery of paternity—something that is not evident in primitive civilizations.

"Since the phallus offers a kinesthetic and visual comparison to the serpent and fish, we might expect some storied recognition of the comparison, as was noted by the Abbé Breuil. Since the phallus was involved in the ejection of semen and urine, we might expect some storied explanation of these processes, which could compare with the vulval connection to menstrual blood. None of these stories concerning masculine processes need involve the female, nor include a knowledge of insemination or fertilization. They could be part of a specialized masculine mythology, perhaps told at the initiation of boys or at a convocation of hunters or as part of the male shaman's repertory" (Alexander Marshack, *The Roots of Civilization*, pp. 330–32).

Beginning with the Magdalenian epoch (about 13,000 B.C. to about 6000 B.C.) representations of the phallus multiplied. The site of Audoubert in the Pyrenees is covered with engraved phalluses. In Placard (old Magdalenian) a bone has been found on which a phallus was carved with a stream of liquid leaving the meatus. It is similar to those of successive epochs, such as the phallic baton of Bruniquel (Dordogne) or the double phallus of the Gorge d'Enfer.

From Eyzies (later Magdalenian) comes a carved bone depicting the head of a bear, with its mouth open, facing a phallus whose testicles resemble flowers. Myth and tradition associate the image of the phallus to fish, water, and serpents.

A fish is carved on the Gorge d'Enfer phallus. In Placard the eyes of the fish have the form of testicles. In Bruniquel can be found one phallic fish after another, all very realistic, with waves representing water. In the grotto of the Trois Frères, in Ariège, there are representations of masked, horned ithyphallic men wearing beast skins, who are very likely shamans, wizards, or dancers.

India is the only region where the cult of the lingam—the phallus—

as well as its rituals and legendary narratives has been perpetuated without interruption from prehistory to the present day. It is thanks to Indian documents, therefore, that we are able to understand the reasons justifying the existence of this cult, the philosophical conceptions that explain it, and the significance of the legends whose variants, as we will see, are to be found everywhere.

The cult of the ithyphallic god of the protohistorical civilization of India was unknown to the Aryan invaders who came out of the north about the third millennium previous to our own era. The phallus cult has no place in Vedic rituals. The god-phallus (Shisna-deva) is, however, mentioned in the *Rig Veda* (7.12.5, and 10.99.3) as well as in the *Nirukta* (4.29), but its worship is banned.

It is the same in the Greco-Roman world where phallic cults came from civilizations predating the arrival of the Achaeans. "A colossal rough image of the ithyphallic god Min [dates] from predynastic Egypt (circa 4500 B.C.)" (Rawson, *Primitive Erotic Art*, p. 14).

The conflict between the ancient cult of Shiva, the ithyphallic god of Nature, and the social religion of the Aryan or Semite invaders is illustrated in the stories of the Purānas, the "ancient chronicles" of Shaivism.

According to the *Shiva Purāna (Rudra Samhitā, Satī Khānda,* 1.22–23), the patriarch Daksha, who is preparing a Vedic sacrifice, is cursed by Nandi (Joyous), the bull, the animal kingdom's companion and personification of Shiva, whose symbol is the phallus. Nandi speaks of Daksha with disdain:

"This ignorant mortal hates the sole god who remains benevolent towards his detractors, and he refuses to recognize the truth. He concerns himself with naught but his domestic life and all the compromises which that entails. To satisfy his interests he practices interminable rituals with a mentality debased by Vedic prescriptions. He forgets the nature of the soul, as he is preoccupied with something totally different. The brutal Daksha, who thinks only of his women, will henceforth have the head of a goat. May this stupid individual, swollen with the vanity he takes in his own knowledge, as well as all those who with him oppose the Great Archer Shiva, continue to dwell in their ignorant ritualism.

"May these enemies of 'He who soothes suffering,' whose spirit is troubled by the odor of the sacrifices and flowery phrases of the Vedas, continue to dwell in their illusions. May all these priests who think only of eating, who put no stake in knowledge save that which profits them, that practice abstinence and ceremonies only to earn a living, seeking naught but wealth and honors, end up as beggars."

The vedic sage Bhrigu, who presides at the sacrifice, replies:

"All those who practice the rites of Shiva and follow him are only heretics who oppose the true faith. They have renounced ritual purity. They dwell in error. Their hair is tangled, and they wear necklaces of bones. They coat themselves in ashes. They practice the initiation rites of Shiva in which intoxicating liquors are considered sacred beverages. Since they scorn the Vedas and the Brahmans, the supports of the social order, they are heretics. The Vedas are the sole path of virtue. Thus let them follow their god, the king of evil spirits."

Despite this antagonism, Shaivism and the lingam cult were incorporated little by little into the Vedic religion as well as into numerous philosophical texts and legendary tales related to it. However, the whole of the texts coming from pre-Aryan culture and banned by the invaders were translated into their language, Sanskrit, and published only after the revival of Shaivism, starting about the second century B.C.

Corsica: Standing stones in phallic form, 3000 B.C. Photograph by Louis Trémellat.

The oldest images of the ithyphallic god and the phallus in India come from the civilization of Mohenjo Daro (two or three millennia before our time). The megalithic monuments found in India and Europe, however, are even older.

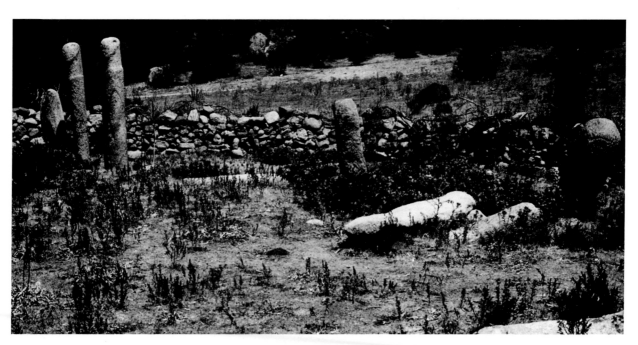

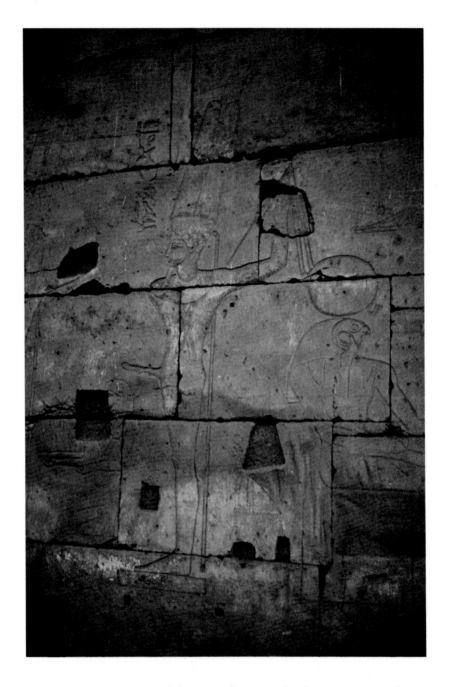

The European megalithic complex precedes the Aegean contribution and the sexual significance of the menhirs is universally attested to.... the belief in the fertilizing virtues of the menhirs was still shared by European peasants at the beginning of the century.... The megalithic complex would have radiated out from one sole center, very likely the eastern Mediterranean . . . linked to Tantricism. . . . Stonehenge (before 2100 B.C.) is pre-Myceanean" (Mircea Eliade, *Histoire des croyances et des idées religieuses,* pp. 130 and 135).

Egypt: Glyph showing Pharaoh's power of procreation, Temple of Karnak exterior wall. Luxor. Photograph by Jeanie Levitan.

Historical Sources

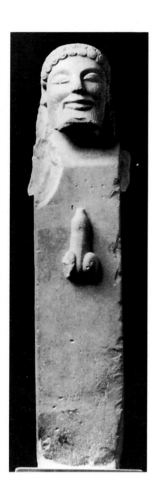

Greece: Hermes of Siphnos. Marble. National Museum, Athens. Photograph by Antonia Mulas.

We have discovered the worship of the phallus in both Mediterranean and northern Europe from prehistory to the Dionysian cults of the sixth century A.D. The phallus was worshiped in Egyptian temples. In Greece it played a large role in the ceremonies honoring Hermes and Dionysus. In Egypt special honors were given to the sex of the butchered Osiris. The worship of the sacred foreskin, brought back from Palestine by Godefroy of Bouillon and still practiced in France and Italy, is a vestige of this cult. One can see erect phalluses on tombs in Anatolia, in Phrygia from the pre-Hellenic epoch, and in Italy dating from the first Iron Age. In Rome, "the custom of sculpting a phallus on the walls of the city comes from the Etruscans" (Jean Mercadé, *Roma Amor*). This is also the case for the Roman *bulla*, a phallic amulet carried by Roman generals on the days commemorating their victories.

In the Greek world, Orpheus was originally considered a native of Thrace, where one phallus cult originated. Hermes was revered under the form of Priapus by a column crowned with a head and decorated with a sex organ.

"One of the most basic of Celtic god-types . . . is the horned, phallic god of the Celtic tribes. . . . The earliest Celtic portrayal of the antlered god occurs in the ancient sanctuary in the Val Camonica in northern Italy . . . round about 400 B.C. The antlered god is known from one inscription only as Cernunnos, 'The Horned One.' . . . Over his left, bent arm are traces of the horned serpent, his most consistent cult animal. . . . his worshipper, smaller in size and having his hands raised in the same *orans* posture as the god—a posture used by the Celts for prayer—is markedly ithyphallic. . . . Sometimes, in Roman contexts, the horned god was likened to Mercury, no doubt in his earlier role as the protector of the flocks and herds. Here too he is usually ithyphallic, but carries instead of weapons the purse and wand of the classical god" (Anne Ross, in *Primitive Erotic Art,* pp. 83–84).

◆

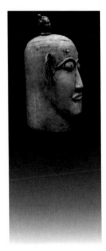

2

◆

SYMBOLISM

THE IMAGE OF THE WORLD'S CREATOR

The means by which a male infant is distinguished at birth is his sex organ. It is why the masculine organ is called in Sanskrit *lingam*—a word that implies "sign."

"The distinctive sign by which one can recognize the nature of something is therefore called lingam" (*Linga Purāna,* 1.6.106).

The principle from which the universe has issued is formless, without lingam, without a distinctive sign.

"Shiva (the supreme divinity) is without sign (without sex), without color, without taste, without odor, beyond the reach of words or touch, without qualities, immutable and immobile" (*Linga Purāna,* 1.3.2–3).

Absolute being, not being manifested, can be perceived only by means of its creation, which is its sign—its lingam. The existence of a transcendent being who *thinks* the world can be known only through this sign. The lingam, or phallus, the source of life, is the form by which the Absolute Being, from whom the world is issued, can be evoked.

"We revere in the sun the dispenser of light, the sum of all eyes; it is in the same regard that in the phallus we worship Shiva who is present

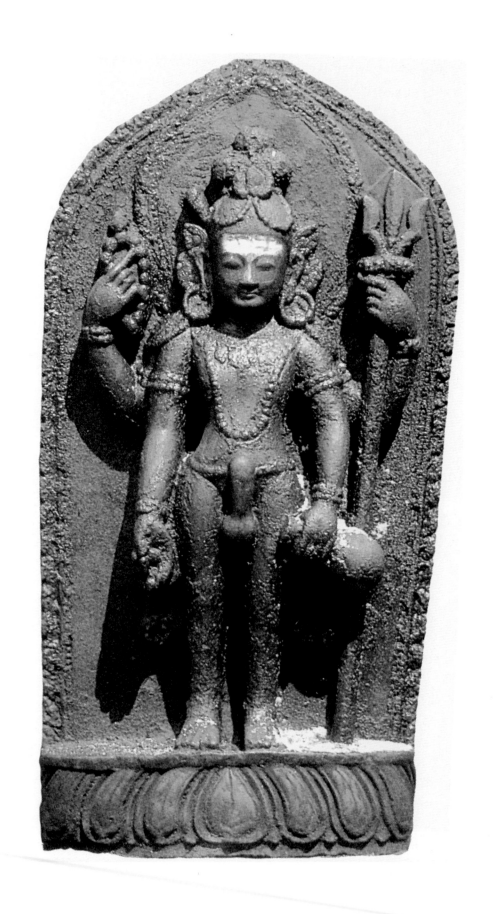

in all generative power. It is not one particular eye that we venerate and make images of, but the sun, the complete eye that gives us sight, the sun that is the source of all visibility. In the same regard it is Shiva, the total being, who is revered in the phallus, his symbol" ("Lingopāsanā Rahasya," *Siddhanta*, vol. 2, p. 154).

"By worshiping the lingam one is not deifying a physical organ, but simply recognizing a form that is eternal and divine manifested in the microcosm. The human organ is the image of the divine emblem, the eternal and causal form of the lingam, present in all things. The phallus is the perceptible aspect of the divinity who exceeds the state of noncreation by the width of ten fingers" *(Purusha Sūkta)*.

In the microcosm, which is to say in man, the sexual organ, the source of life, is the form in which the nature of the formless manifests itself. However, "it is not the phallus in itself which is revered but that for which it is the sign—the progenitor, the cosmic individual. The phallus is the emblem, the sign of the individual Shiva for whom it is the symbol" (*Shiva Purāna*, 1.16.106–7).

"The symbol of the cosmic man Purusha, the archetype, the universal plan present in all things, is the male emblem, the phallus. The symbol of energy, which is the world's substance, the generator of all that exists, is the female organ, the yoni" ("Lingopāsanā Rahasya," p. 154).

THE SYMBOL OF THE UNIVERSE

In the being without form within which exists no distinctive sign appears a sign which is the Universe. This sign can be mentioned, touched, breathed, seen, and tasted. It is the source of both coarse and subtle elements" (*Linga Purāna*, 1.3.3–4).

"Fundamental Nature is therefore called phallus. He who possesses this distinctive sign is the supreme being" (*Linga Purāna* 1.17.5).

"The lingam has its roots in the formless, in the nonmanifested (avyakta). Shiva is therefore in himself without the lingam. The lingam is the thing-of-Shiva" (*Linga Purāna* 1.3.3–4).

"Shiva, as an indivisible causal principle, is worshiped under the form of the phallus. His different manifestations within the created world are represented by anthropomorphic images. All the other gods form part of the multiplicity and are therefore represented by images" ("Shrī Shiva Tattva," *Siddhānta*).

OPPOSITE
Nepal: Ithyphallic Shiva, seventeenth century. Kathmandu. Photograph by Ira Landgarten from James Wasserman's Art and Symbols of the Occult *(Destiny Books).*

Symbolism

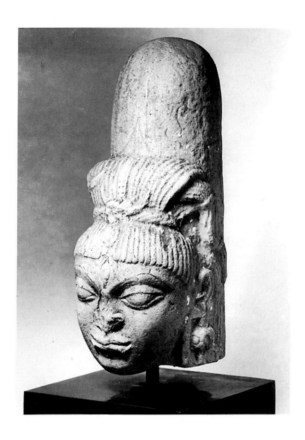

India: White crystalline sandstone Shiva lingam, circa fourth century. Photograph by Nik Douglas.

"In the hierarchy of the created, it is the sun that appears as the progenitor of the terrestrial world. It is the image of the creator, which is why its symbol is the organ of procreation" (*Shiva Purāna*, 1.16.105).

"Shiva said: I am not distinct from the phallus. The phallus is identical to me. It draws my faithful close to me; therefore it must be worshiped. My beloveds! Everywhere an erect penis is to be found I am present, even if it is no more than another of my representations" (*Shiva Purāna*, 1.9.43–4).

"The entire world has the phallus as its foundation. All is issued from the lingam. He who desires perfection of the soul must worship the lingam" (*Linga Purāna*, 1.3.7).

"It is the lord who is the source of all pleasure.... For existence to be a perpetual joy, the faithful should worship the phallus, which is Shiva himself. We venerate the sun which gives birth to the world and sustains it as the symbol of the origin of the terrestrial world. In the same regard, it is under the form of the phallus that Shiva, the universal principle, should be revered. This is why the male principle is recognizable as that which is called phallus. The phallus is the symbol of the god" (*Shiva Purāna*, 1.16.103–6).

THE MAHĀ-LINGAM,
OR TRANSCENDENT SIGN

"Purusha, the cosmic man (the ideational principle of the world) and Prakriti, Nature (the universal substance) are one and yet distinct and, even though distinct, inseparable. They exist only by their relationship to each other. From the perspective of principle, they form part of manifestation; from the perspective of the world, however, they exist before creation. It is their nondivisible state, the stage at which the sign, the lingam, is still united to that which is without sign (alingam), which is called the transcendental sign: the Mahā-lingam. It represents the independent divinity (niralamba) beyond change (nirvikāra)" (Gopinātha Kavirāj, "Linga Rahasya," *Kalyāna*, Shiva anka, p. 476).

"Universal Consciousness, which is the first stage in the order of creation, is called *mahat*, the 'great principle.' It forms the womb in which I deposit my semen. From it comes, according to the hierarchy of creation, all elements and all creatures" (*Bhagavad Gītā*, 14.3).

"To the Latin philosophers and mythographers, the god Pan, represented by Priapus, is the symbol of the Whole, of the Universe. In the Orphic litanies, Pan is the first principle of love, the creator incorporated into universal matter. Sky, earth, fire, and water are its limbs" (Payne Knight, *The Worship of Priapus*, p. 13).

DIVINE EROS

Within the immutable causal being first appears desire, the desire to procreate. "He will desire. May I procreate! May I exist for always!" (*Taittrīya Upanishad*, 2.6.1). In Greece, Eros is always associated with Himeros, desire.

"Desire, the attraction of opposites, is the first manifestation of dualism; it gives birth to the distinction between the person and Nature. Tied to Nature by desire, the cosmic person procreates countless worlds. This desire, this inclination to pleasure, that makes up part of his nature, is supernatural Eros" (Karpātri, "Lingopāsanā Rahasya," p. 153).

"Desire forms part of the universal Being, which is present in all things" (*Bhāgavata Purāna*, 10.55.1).

"Born from the primordial egg, Eros was the first of the gods; none of the others could have been born without him. Born before

Symbolism

Aphrodite, he is the origin of all species of plants and animals. He is responsible for the union of Heaven and Earth.

"To Orphism, Eros Protogonos, the primordial principle of Eros, appeared at the same time as the Ether, which is to say at the beginning of the world. Child of time (Kronos) and necessity (Anagyn), he acts upon inert matter (Chaos), eternally engendering.

"In the Orphic hymns, Eros is the 'father of the night,' attracting light unto himself. He penetrates the world by the movement of his wings. He is called the Magnificent, the Sovereign, Priapus, the Illuminated One" (Payne Knight, *The Worship of Priapus*, p. 9).

"[Eros] was a wild boy, who showed no respect for age or station but flew about on golden wings, shooting barbed arrows at random or wantonly setting hearts on fire with his dreadful torches. . . . His most famous shrine was at Thespiae, where the Boeotians worshipped him as a simple phallic pillar—the pastoral Hermes, or Priapus, under a different name" (Robert Graves, *The Greek Myths*, I.15.1).

THE PHALLUS, ORGAN OF BLISS

From the mystical Shaivite perspective, as in the Dionysian orgy, erotic ecstasy is only secondarily a means of reproduction. Above all it is a search for pleasure. In erotic rituals, "to please the lord his symbol must be worshiped independently of its physical function. As this function is to give birth, that function is thereby excluded" (*Shiva Purāna*, 1.16.108).

The union of Shiva and his lovers—Shakti, Pārvatī, or Satī—is not procreative. Their respective infants are engendered separately. Skanda, the god of beauty and the head of the army of gods, was born from the sperm of Shiva, which fell into the mouth of a sacrificial fire and then into the waters of the Ganges. Ganapati, the elephant-headed god who is prayed to at the start of all endeavors and who protects the entrance to the home, is the son of a goddess who formed him from her skin's flakings while she bathed.

"According to the *Sefer Yezirah*, the phallus fulfills a function that is not only generational but confers equilibrium in regard to the structures built by man and the order of the world. For that reason the connection was established between this 'seventh member' and the

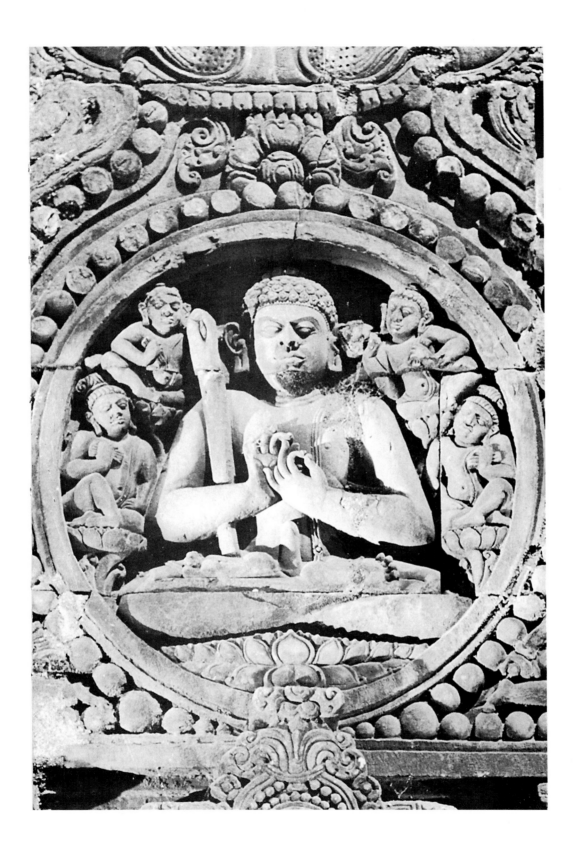

righteous seventh day of creation. Under various representations it designates the creative force and it is worshiped as the very source of life" (G. C. Scholem, *Les Origines de la Kabbale*, pp. 164–65).

Pleasure, in the Shaivite conception, is the image of the divine state. This is why, when the divine manifests itself in its procreative aspect, it shows its aspect as pleasure in equal degree. The sexual organ therefore has a double role: the inferior one of procreation and the superior one of contacting the divine state by means of the ecstasy caused by pleasure (ānanda). The orgasm is a "divine sensation." So whereas paternity attaches man to the things of the earth, the ecstasy of pleasure can reveal divine reality to him, leading him to detachment and spiritual realization. "The phallus is the source of pleasure. It is the sole means of obtaining earthly pleasure and salvation. By looking at it, touching it, and meditating on it, living beings are capable of freeing themselves from the cycle of future lives" (*Shiva Purāna*, 1.9.20).

"Pleasure's center resides in the sexual organ (upastha), in the cosmic lingam, source of all orgasmic joy. In the terrestrial world, all love, all sensuality, every desire is a quest for that pleasure. We desire things only insofar as they can procure for us sensual bliss. Divinity is only a love object when it represents an unmitigated sensual pleasure. Other things are merely the objects of a temporary love, because they can bring only fleeting satisfactions.

"Lustful desire for women exists only because one sees within it the form of one's own pleasure and the source of enjoyment. The joy of possession momentarily tames the suffering of desire, and man can then experience the pleasure that is his desire's target. Within that pleasure he perceives his own essential nature, which is joy.

"Every orgasm, every pleasure is a divine experience. The entire universe springs forth from enjoyment. Pleasure is at the origin of all that exists. But the perfect love is that whose object is limitless. It is that love which is pure love, love of love itself, the love of the transcendental being-of-sensual-pleasure" (Karpatri, "Lingopāsanā Rahasya," p. 153).

BĪJA, THE SEMEN

Sperm is the essence of life, the best of oblations, the purest form of sacrificial elixir (soma). All beings are born from an offering of sperm hurled into the fire of desire. There is a representation of Agni, lord of

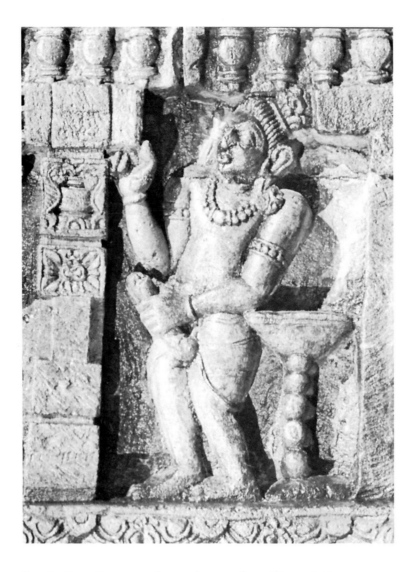

fire, drinking the sperm that gushes out from Shiva's phallus.

Sperm is worshiped under various names. It fills the cup of the moon worn by Shiva on his forehead. It is the Ganges flowing from the head of the lingam. All forms of oblation and all beverages that give life or immortality are represented as forms of Shiva's sperm.

Sperm is called *bīja* (the semen), *soma* (the oblation), *chandra* (the moon), and *virya* (the virile essence). "In Egypt the sun god Re-Atum-Khepri manufactured all of creation by masturbating" (Mircea Eliade, *Histoire des croyances et des idées religieuses*, p. 101).

The sex organ is that mysterious organ through which the creative principle is manifested by giving birth to a new being. It is therefore the organ by which that principle is visibly represented in every particular species. Sperm, which potentially contains the entire ancestral

India: Temple of Gyaraspur. Bas-relief known as "sperm sacrifice on the domestic altar," eighth century.

Symbolism

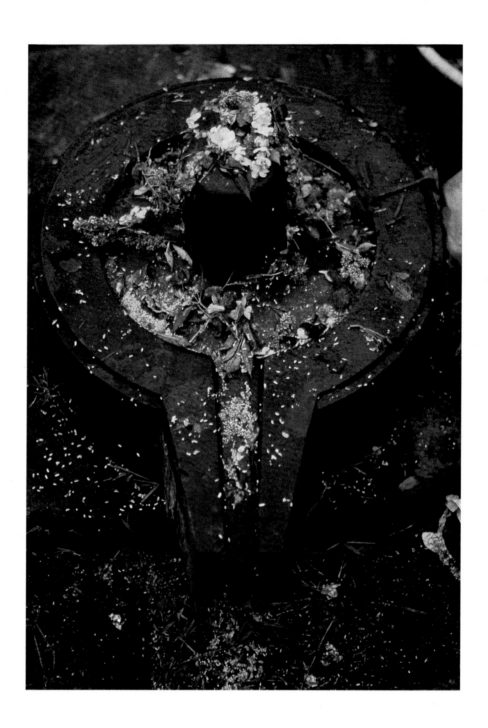

Nepal: Shiva lingam with pilgrims' offerings. Kathmandu. Photograph by Kevin Bubriski.

heritage, race, and characteristics of the person to be, is called *bindu* (point limit). Indeed, it is the minute passage between being and nonbeing. The sex organ is thereby that organ by which communication is established between man and the creative force, the manifestation of the divine being.

Within the microcosm, which is to say within man, the design is contained within the semen and becomes real only through the matter that nourishes it within the belly of the mother—the egg, which is the departure point of all living things.

Ritual offerings of sperm were part of agrarian rites in various civilizations. Even today, in certain regions of Africa, young men of various tribes dig holes in the earth into which to pour their sperm. In Hindu rites, except in the case of certain tantric practices, symbolic substitutes for sperm are used, such as rainwater and the seeds of rice or grains. "Since the fluid semen came to be identified as the generic cause of fertility, it may well be that the identification of the sky as male, moistening and fertilizing a female earth, which appears in the oldest layers of so many literatures, took place during the very early stages of agriculture" (Philip Rawson, *Primitive Erotic Art*, p. 50).

In alchemy, the origin of which is Shaivite, mercury corresponds to the moon, Shiva's cup of sperm. In tantric ritual the lingam is consecrated with mercury. To the Chinese, who call it liquid silver, mercury represents sperm, water, kidneys, blood, and the dragon. The alternation of mercury with cinnabar corresponds to yin and yang.

In Egypt and Greece, as in India, ritual phalluses are painted with cinnabar. In Western alchemy metals are believed to be produced by the underground conjunction of mercury, considered as feminine semen, and sulfur, considered as masculine semen.

"The semen of Shiva and his lover Satī fell upon the back of the earth and filled the world. It is that seed which caused the appearance of every phallic emblem of Shiva that can be found in the infernal regions, the Earth, and Heaven. From it all past and future emblems of Shiva are made. Shiva's lingam issued from the radiation of two semens" (*Nārada Pañcharātra*, 3.1).

THE VULVA (YONI)

In the sanctuary where it is worshiped, the lingam is represented surrounded by the female organ, the yoni.

"Universal energy, the substance of the world, is represented by the yoni, which grasps the lingam. It is only when the phallus, the giver of semen, is surrounded by the yoni that God can manifest and the universe appear.

"The symbol of the cosmic man, Purusha, the formless, the immutable, the all-seeing eye, is the masculine emblem, the phallus. The symbol of the energy that is the world's substance, generator of all that exists, is represented by the female organ, the yoni" (Karpātri, "Lingopāsanā Rahasya," p. 154). "The yoni represents the womb of the visible and the subtle world" (*Yajur Veda, Vājasenīya Samhitā*, 13.3; *Taittirīya Samhitā* 4.2.8.2), "the universal womb in which all things that are individual develop" (*Shvetāshvatara Upanishad*, 5.55).

The phallus fertilizes that womb. The semen giver is the phallus; it fertilizes Nature, giving birth to the visible world and to the multiple forms of life.

"Because it is the origin of all life, nature is comparable to a womb" (*Shiva Purāna*, 1.16.101).

"This womb is Nature, the base of all existence. He that sports with her is Shiva. It is he who dispenses pleasure. There is not nor has there ever been any other dispenser" (*Shiva Purāna*, 1.16.101).

As the universal fertilizing principle the phallus is unique. But every form of existence requires a different womb to be fertilized. That is why all the different species are called wombs, or yoni. The Purānas speaks of 8,400,000 yoni, or different species residing on the earth.

The principle called Shiva represents the totality of procreative power to be found in the universe. All individual procreation is a fragment of it.

"The universe is the issue of the relationship between a masculine and a feminine principle. Everything, as a result, carries the signature of the lingam and the yoni. It is the deity who, in the form of the individual phallus, penetrates each womb and procreates all beings" (Karpātri, "Lingopāsanā Rahasya," p. 163).

"It is he alone who actually penetrates every womb" (*Shvetāshvatara Upanishad*, 5.2).

The very name *Delphi* stems from *delphys*: womb.

THE UNION OF THE SEXES

In the state preceding embodiment, the gods form but one sole being; there is no perceptible duality, no positive or negative force. But from the moment that the first tendency towards manifestation appears in the nondifferentiated substratum, duality is already present. This duality has the character of two poles of opposite attraction—one of positive tendency, the other negative—which are manifested throughout creation under male and female aspects. There is no possibility of creation without the union of opposites. Nothing can issue from either Shiva or Nature alone. For creation to take place, the union of an active and a passive principle, a male organ and a female organ, is indispensable. The union of the cosmic person and universal Nature is represented by the copulation *(maithuna)* of Shiva and the goddess.

Transcendental virility is the immanent cause of creation. Transcendental femininity is its efficient cause. These principles, in the microcosm, are especially apparent in the reproductive organs, which represent the essential physical function of all living beings. In nature everything pivots on reproduction and is made to assure the continuity of life. It is in the union of the lingam and the yoni that divinity, the power to create, becomes visible in man. Procreation is impossible without such a union, and divine manifestation is equally so without its cosmic equivalent.

The rituals that provide the means for us to communicate with the gods are interwoven with the act of making love.

"The first appeal is the invocation of the god *(hinkāra).*

"The invitation represents the laudes *(prastāra).*

"Sleeping next to the woman is the magnificat *(udgītha).*

"Facing one another is the choir *(pratihāra).*

"The orgasm is the consecration.

"Separation is the closing hymn *(nidhāna).*

"He who understands that every sexual act is a hymn addressed to Vama-deva, the fiery form of Shiva, recreates himself with each copulation. He will thrive all the days of his life; he will live long and become wealthy in both offspring and in livestock; rich will be his renown" *(Chāndogya Upanishad*, 2.13.1).

In Celtic mythology there is "the powerful Fergus mac Roich, 'Fergus son of Great Horse', the name itself being suggestive of virility. . . . His penis is described as being seven fingers in length; he mates with the divine queen Medb, 'Drunk Woman', whose own sexuality is boundless" (Anne Ross, in *Primitive Erotic Art*, p. 83).

The transmission of the genetic code and its transplanting into a rigorously selected soil, the transfer to a new being of an ancestral heritage containing the archetypes bequeathed it by divine thought, is the most important religious act of a man's life. It must be practiced as a

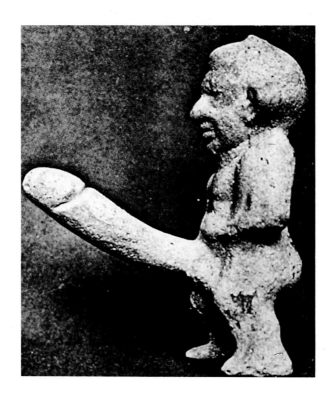

ritual, following rules that take into account the most favorable moments and the convergence of the stars, in such a way that the new flame-bearer is suitably adapted to his role and that the breed fashioned by the long line of ancestors continues and neither is degraded nor dies out in the course of its journey. All religions accord a central role to the act of reproduction in its moral code, even if at times they have lost the true meaning of it and reversed its values. Sexual diversion under any of its myriad forms is not to be condemned, so much as the progeny of ill-matched couples, the blending of breeds or races who deform the model drawn by the gods and transmitted by the ancestral lineage.

Procreation's rituals are described in the Tantras. They include adoration of the genitals as images of the divine principles poised to unite to accomplish the miracle. No longer to view in these organs this image of the divine principle or to revere them as such constitutes the first step toward moral decadence and the degradation of the species.

Only through sexual union are new beings capable of existing. This union, therefore, represents a place between two worlds, a point of contact between being and nonbeing, where life manifests itself and incarnates the divine spirit. The forms of the organs that achieve this ritual are symbolic. They are the visible form of the creator.

THE FATHER, PHALLUS-BEARER

Everything in all living beings—human and animal as well as in the plant kingdom—is centered on the procreative organ. Man is merely the "phallus-bearer" *(linga-dhara)*, the servant of his sexual organ. The idea of God the father is a puritanical transposition of the divine phallus. The father is someone whose sexual organ pours semen into a receptacle, the *argha*, or vagina.

To Freud, the phallus signified this aspect of sexuality that could not be claimed by the individual.

Shiva and his energy, Shakti, envisioned as the source of all manifestation, are symbolized by the procreative organs. The possessor of the phallus represents the unmanifested stage, which remains unknowable. In a less abstract symbolism, the unknowable entity, whose sign is the phallus, can be replaced by the father, the phallus bearer. The total Being, the entity for whom creation is sexual bliss and for whom the phallus is a symbol, is indeed at times called the father.

"O Son of Kunti! Beings born of every womb come from the womb of Immensity, and I am the father, the semen giver."

"I am the father of this world" *(Bhagavad Gītā,* 14.4; 9.17).

"Like a father and a mother, the Being who thinks the world and the matter in which it is realized gives birth to all the forms of existence. In this world, the men who desire progeny impregnate women. In the same fashion, the Supreme Being, desiring a progeny, desiring to multiply itself, impregnates Nature" ("Lingopāsana Rahaysa," p. 153).

It is the function that is both important and permanent. The individual who achieves this duty, who carries the organ, is merely its temporary and interchangeable instrument. The tendency to replace the symbol—the procreative organ—by the figurative image of the father is a substitution that allows the intervention of useless anthropomorphic elements, which diminish the degree of abstraction the divine aspect represents.

For Freud, "sexual reproduction made the individual into a contingent carrier, truly the appendage of the genetic code. The discovery of the phallic phase is equivalent to the recognition of the symbolic order's supremacy in relation to the real and the imaginary . . . the anteriority of the signifier in relation to the signified."

◆

Symbolism

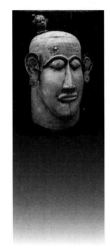

3

◆

REPRESENTATIONS OF THE PHALLUS

THE STANDING STONE

Everywhere the phallus cult spread, its presence is affirmed by the standing stones that can be found from India, Greece, Mesopotamia, Thrace, Crete, Malta, and Corsica to the very edge of Brittany and England.

At Knossos, as in Thebes and Malta, the god was honored in the form of a column. Orthos, the "upstanding," represents Dionysus-pillar or Dionysus-Priapus. Shiva is *urdhva-linga*, "he of the erect penis." He is referred to as Sthānu (column), as Dionysus is called Perikionios (of the column). The Minoan pillars, according to Evans, are nonfigurative images of the deities. Square pillars were representations of Hermes; cylindrical columns, symbols of Mercury.

The phallus is worshiped in the form of a standing stone *(sailaja)* or, more certainly, in the ithyphallic image of a god. It is also represented grasped by the yoni, the female organ, in which form it appears in Shaivite temples.

Shiva's emblem, the phallus, is represented standing vertically in shrines, divided into three sections. The lowest section is squared and concealed within the pedestal. It represents Brahmā, the maker, the gravitational power that shapes worlds. The octagonal central section

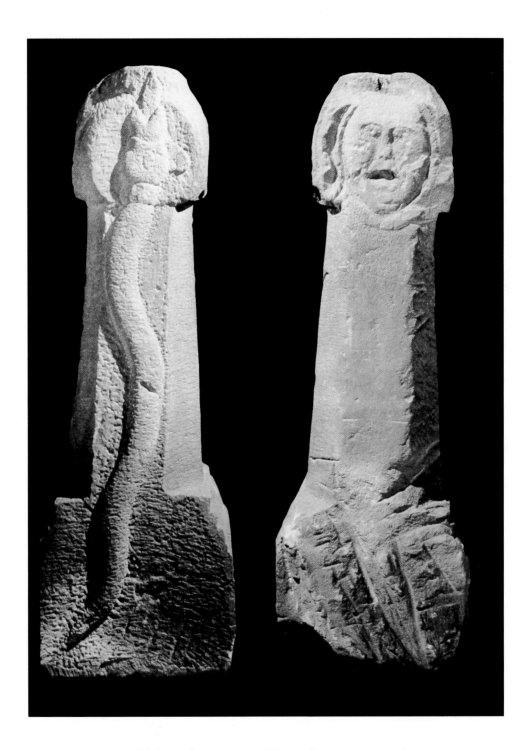

represents Vishnu, the centripetal force of concentration that gives birth to matter. The upper section is cylindrical and represents Shiva, the centrifugal force of expansion that issues forth matter and form from its outpourings. The base of the lingam itself is gripped by the yoni, the receptacle.

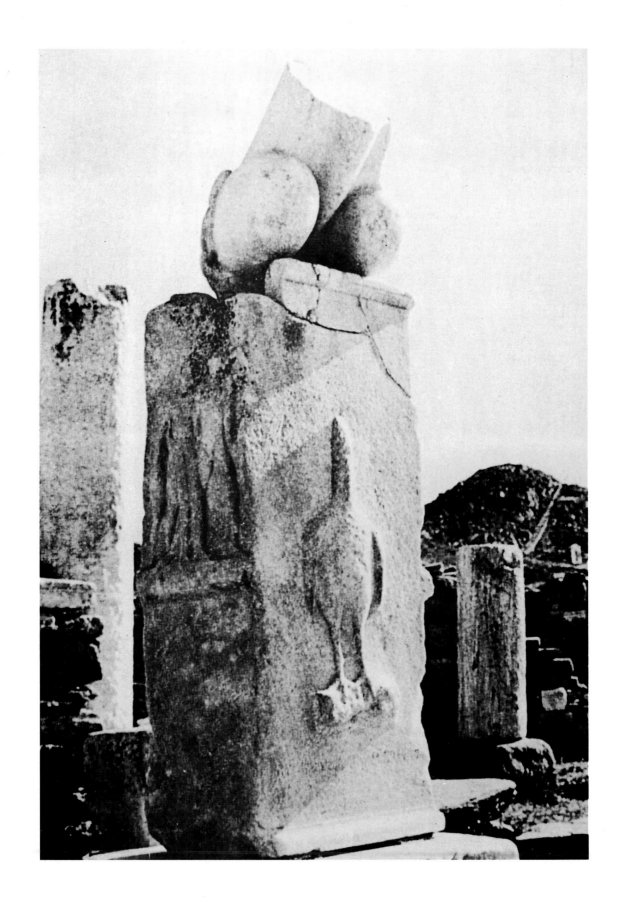

"Brahma is the root, and the center is Vishnu, lord of the three worlds. Rising above at the top is the proud Rudra, the Great God, the eternal Peacegiver whose name is the magic syllable OM [Rudra, the 'howler,' represents that aspect of the creation that remains present in his work]. The altar of the phallus is the Great Goddess. The phallus itself is the true God" (*Linga Purāna*, 1.73.19–20).

The part of the phallus seized by the yoni is creation's source, the First Cause in contact with Nature.

"The Universal Mother forms the altar. The phallus itself represents pure consciousness" (*Shiva Purāna* 1.11.22).

"The largest part of the phallus remains out of Nature's reach, forever withdrawn from the whole of creation" *(Udāsīna).*

"One fourth represents the universe with its elements and all of its beings. The three fourths above are the Immortal One" *(Purusha Sūkta).*

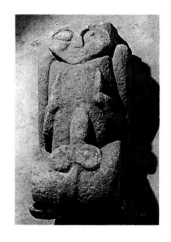

The lingam is placed in the center of the tabernacle, a dark cubical chamber, which is the womb, the *garbagriha* of the temple. The axis of the erect phallus determines how the temple's tower is lined up with its peak. This then evokes the lingam of light, which is the axis of the world.

Large phalluses made of wood, metal, or stone were installed within the Dionysian chapels. The monument in Delos, which dates from the beginning of the Hellenistic era, is formed of a pedestal of quadrangular marble upon which is carved a bird with outstretched claws: the Dionysian bird-phallus. On the other sides are reliefs depicting priests, maidens bearing baskets on their heads, and worshipers. On top of the pedestal stands a phallus, which, though broken today, must have been more than a yard and a half in length. Its testicles were covered with feathers.

Analogous to the phallus through which sperm travels, the pillar appears as a means of communication through which courses the life-giving principle of the sacred. It is the symbol of the tree of life, the world's axis.

In Egypt, Osiris was represented by a pillar called a *djed*.

In Celtic cosmology, the pillar also plays an essential role. The title of the Irish tale announcing the apocalypse is "The Plain of Pillars." Decapitated heads were often placed on menhirs, giving them a close resemblance to the cippi of Hermes.

In Solomon's temple, the right column represented the active male

ABOVE
British Isles: Cave statue of phallic character. Morgan Abbey, Glamorgan. Photograph by C. M. Dixon from Philip Rawson's Primitive Erotic Art *(Weidenfeld & Nicolson).*

OPPOSITE
Greece: Column topped with a phallus. Monument of Karystios in Delos, 300 B.C.

Representations of the Phallus

principle, and the column on the left, the passive female principle. This symbolism has been expropriated by Freemasons. In every Masonic lodge a red painted column on the right represents the male principle, called *J* (Jakin), while on the left a white painted column called *B* (Boaz) invokes the female principle.

The pillar represents the world's axis to Australian aborigines, for whom a ritual pole is evocative of that used by Numbakula, the Creator, to forge the structures of the cosmos.

The installation of a stone phallus, preferably in secluded spots or in the mountains, is a meritorious act. The ancient sanctuaries of Shiva, like those for Dionysius, were located away from cities by preference.

This is also the case for the megaliths in England, Brittany, and Corsica and in the whole world stretching from India to Europe's extreme western borders.

The Egyptian obelisk is a phallic symbol. The same is true of steeples and minarets of later religions, during their earliest manifestations.

"Diodorus of Sicily recalls that Sesostris raised columns representing male organs as a homage to those peoples who bravely defended themselves" (Payne Knight, *The Worship of Priapus*, p. 114).

Votive or triumphal columns, such as the Trajan column erected in Rome as a gesture of gratitude, are also closely tied to the same symbolism.

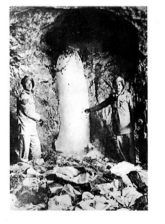

SPONTANEOUS MANIFESTATIONS OF THE SACRED PHALLUS *(SVAYAMBHŪ)*

Given that the creator remains forever present within his own work, objects that evoke the form of the sacred emblem appear spontaneously at times. One such embodiment is to be found in the Amarnatha grotto in Kashmir, where thousands of pilgrims come annually to worship a lingam made of ice.

"The semen of god falls upon the surface of the earth and fills the world. It is this seed that causes the appearance of all the lingams of Shiva to be found throughout the infernal regions, the Earth and Heaven" *(Nārada Pañcharāta).*

Sixty-eight of these *svayambhū* lingams, which today have become cult objects in various regions of India, are important pilgrimage destinations.

In the sacred waters of the Narbada River, in central India, pebbles called *shālagrāma* can be found that are evocative of the phallic form.

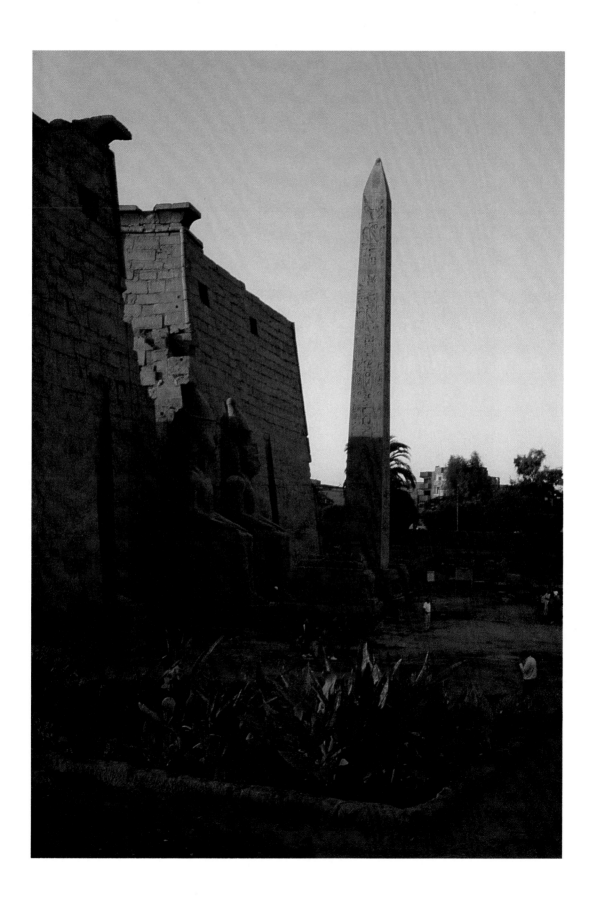

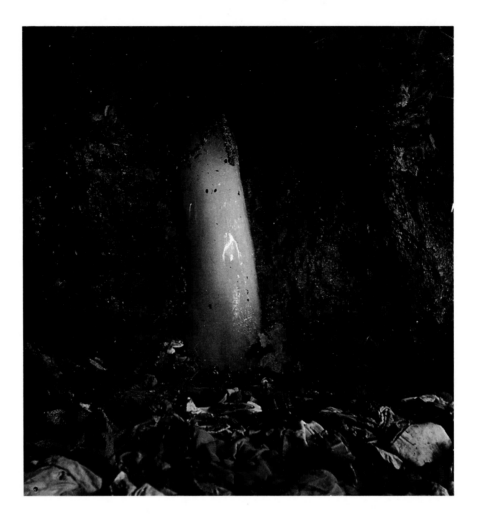

They are dearly sought after and are collected and adored by numerous Hindus.

SHAPELESS OBJECTS (BETHELS)

Sometimes the presence of God can be felt in apparently shapeless objects, which are therefore considered lingams. This is the case of the rough stone, adored under the name of Eros, that Pausanias (9.27.1) saw in Thespia, and also of the black rock of Mecca, the Makheshvara of the ancient Hindus.

Bethel, a term of Semitic origin (beith-El) meaning "the house of God," is the contemporary appellation for those sacred stones worshiped in Arab countries, before Islam, as so many receptacles of divine potency. Such stones served also as cult centers for the ancient Hebrews. Their worship was considered idolatrous by Moses, who ordered their destruction (Leviticus 26:1, Numbers 33:52).

With his head resting on such a stone, however, Jacob received in a dream the revelation of his descendants' destiny (Genesis 28:11–19). He erected a monument of this stone, which became a place of pilgrimage. In equal measure, Joshua erected a stone as testimony of his pact with Jehovah (Joshua 24:27).

Ireland's main idol was called Cromm Cruaich or Fallstone and was surrounded by a dozen other menhirs. St. Patrick, who put an end to this cult, struck them with his cross, causing them to sink into the earth. At Kemaria, in the Morbihan area, a bethel that no longer exists was marked with a swastika.

In Thespia, Eros was worshiped in the form of a bethel until Praxiteles sculpted an image of him in the fourth century B.C. The talking stones utilized by oracles are often aerolites, such as the black stone of Cybele, the Trojan statue of Pallas Athena, and that which the Dalai Lama receives from the king of the world.

THE OMPHALOS

The omphalos is a white phallic stone, rounded at the top, which represents the center of the world. It is the throne of a superhuman presence. The cosmic omphalos, which represents the male principle, is the opposite of the cosmic egg, which signifies the female principle. The omphalos appears most frequently surrounded by snakes, similar to the Indian lingam, thereby evoking the union of the sexes.

The omphalos of Delphi was the center of the cult of Apollo. It was situated, according to Varron, on the spot where Apollo slew the serpent Python. According to Pindar, it was not merely the center of the world but the center of the universe. It represented the means of communication between the three worlds. Certain menhirs are also omphalos.

"Aigeus is a term signifying a pointed or conical pillar. According to Hesychios, it was an altar in the form of a pillar erected in front of an entrance.... The cult of Aigeus, principally but not exclusively associated with Apollo, sprang from the Aigeus pillar cult linked to Minoan pillar worship. The cult of the sacred stone, guardian of roads and portals, which was the essential aspect of Aigeus in ancient Greece, existed in earlier times in Anatolia. The label *Aigeus*, normally considered to be a reference to Apollo, was also attributed to Zeus and Dionysus. This is a clear indication that the cult of the standing stone was earlier than its association with Apollo" (R. F. Willets, *Cretan Cults and Festivals,* pp. 259–60).

The black stone of Heliopolis, in ancient Egypt, bore the name of *benben* (from the root *bn,* to gush forth), which is reminiscent of the Indian *skanda* (the jet of sperm). The benben was the image of the primordial hill upon which the god Atoum had created the first couple. The black stone of Cybele, the conical image of the mountain, was itself also an omphalos. The pyramid and the obelisk are evocative of the original benben, with its ties to the omphalos and the cult of the phallus. The cornerstone of the Ark of the Covenant in Jerusalem, ever visible near Christ's tomb, was an omphalos.

In Hebrew tradition, in the *Sepher Bahir,* the phallus is compared to the righteous, who, like a column, are both the foundation and the support that insures equilibrium between Heaven and Earth. Life rests upon a phallus just as the universe rests upon a column.

Cairns, heaps of stones placed at crossroads in the Celtic world, were representations of their central mountain and are another form of the omphalos.

THE PILLAR OF LIGHT

The principle known as Shiva can be represented as the axis of the world as it develops from its point-limit, the *bindu,* the point of departure for the Universe. This world axis is represented as an endless pillar of light—a lingam of light that traverses the universe from one side to the other and is visible to those who have attained a transcendental level of perception.

According to the Purāna, the gods Brahmā and Vishnu were quarreling one day over which of them was the greater. There suddenly appeared before them an immense column of light. Mounted on his swan, Brahmā flew upward, seeking its peak, while Vishnu, in the form of a wild boar, descended to seek its foundation. For thousands of years they were incapable of reaching the column's extremities. Finally they saw a *ketaki* (pandanus) flower that had fallen from the lingam's head. The flower told them, "For ten eons I've been falling and none knows how much more time it will take me to descend and reach the ground."

In yoga, the foundation center at the base of the spinal column is called the hearth, or yoni. Its form is that of the female organ. The igneous force curled up at its heart rises and climbs the length of the path of its realization. This uncoiled energy is then called the lingam of light.

"In the midst of the subtle center situated at the body's lowest point, said to be a triangle whose three sides are desire, knowledge, and action, rises that lingam born of its self and glowing like a thousand suns" *(Shiva Purāna)*.

All bodies' centers are yonis in equal measure, and each has in its core an erect phallus representing the power to know that is present in all things.

THE LINGAM OF SPACE (AKĀSHA LINGAM)

Space is the lingam; the earth is its yoni. Within it dwell all the gods. It is the "sign ," because all dissolves into it *(Skanda Purāna)*.

The vault of the sky appears as an immense phallus rising over the feminine earth. This is the reason that openings in the earth are considered to be wombs, feminine organs, yonis. From this stems the sacred character of caverns and gulfs, of galleries that penetrate deeply into the belly of the Earth Mother. In these wombs are practiced those rituals that assure the fertility and prosperity of harvests and procreation.

All sanctuaries dedicated to the goddess are to be found in grottos. The underground shrines of prehistory, like the later ones of Crete and Malta, are well known. Even in our day, it is within a grotto that the goddess of Lourdes is embodied.

MUKHA LINGAM (PHALLUS WITH A FACE)

For the same reason that a temple roof is retiled with gold, the god emblems are sometimes recovered in a golden screed. Included in this screed, called a *kavacha,* are the armor, certain symbolic elements of the anthropomorphic image of the god, the three eyes, and the lunar crescent—the crown that evokes its majesty to be supreme over all beings and all other gods. The screed permits the transformation of the naked lingam to the lingam with a face *(mukha lingam)*.

Raised phalluses with a face, like those seen in Erma, are to be found throughout the Western world, as in Greece and India. The Celts erected phallic stones with a face carved on the gland. The "face of glory" *(kirti-mukha)* that is found above the shrines in Shaivite

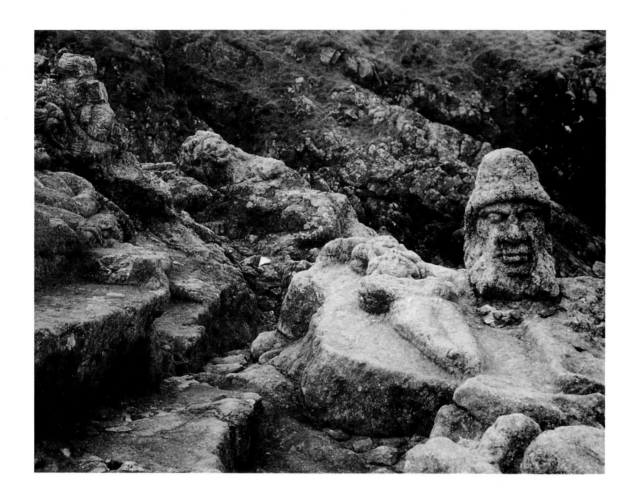

France. Phallus-like monumental head. Rotheneuf.

temples is an elaborate form of the same symbol. From the mouth of this "glory face" situated at the top of the phallic column the entire universe issues forth.

On certain images a complete human figure appears built into the phallic pillar. In southern India, the *gundimallum-lingam* bearing such a figure has been worshiped continuously from the second century B.C. Similar images occurred in medieval Europe.

THE SOVEREIGN OF THE DIRECTIONS OF SPACE, THE PHALLUS OF FIVE FACES

At times the screed is comprised of five faces *(pañcha-mukha lingam)*. These faces represent those aspects of the god that regulate the directions in space and the zenith. These aspects of Shiva linked to the directions are tied in equal measure to the elements as well as to the senses of perception and action of living beings.

Tat-purusha, the regent of matter, is to be found in the east. It corresponds to the element of Earth, the color yellow, sexual bliss, the sense of smell, and the anus.

Aghora, the guardian, governs the south. It corresponds to the element of Ether, the color blue-black, language, intelligence, the sense of hearing, and the ear.

The regent Vāma, god of the left hand and magic, is in the west. It corresponds to the element of Fire, the color red, the ego or the concept of individuality, the power of sight, and the eye.

Sadyojāta, the spontaneous gush, can be found in the north. It corresponds to the element Water, the color white, the intellect, the oblation (sperm, soma), the sense of taste, and the penis.

Ishāna, the Lord, or the transcendent aspect of god (Mahā-deva), can be found at the zenith. It corresponds to the element of Air. It is as colorless as crystal or of a tan color. It represents the coordinator, knowledge, the sense of touch, and the hand.

These concepts are fundamentally important. We will discover, over and over again, their application in every tradition governing the construction of shrines, astrology, the interpretation of omens, yoga postures, the positioning of participants in ceremonial rituals, and other such practices.

Shiva is the ruler of the universe. His different aspects are linked to the deities who rule over the directions of space and to whom an important symbolism is attributed as well as a direct and immediate effect on life. The symbolism of directions can be found in Crete and Egypt, in megalithic cultures, and in Greek and Roman religions, right up through the time of medieval Christianity.

In the *Ajax* of Sophocles, Pan is invoked as the director of the dance of the gods, that is to say, the movements of the universe.

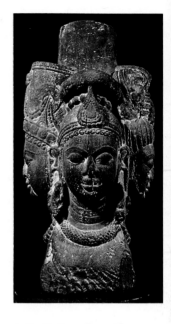

India: Pink sandstone Shiva lingam, circa sixth century. Photograph by Nik Douglas.

THE COSMIC EGG

Totality is often represented in the form of an egg. The universe appears to man as an egg divided in two halves: the earth and the sky. The egg is considered the origin of life. In it the male and the female principles are reunited. The form of the egg is also a sign, a lingam.

In the Tantra, the usual symbol for Shiva is always a phallus, but in the Purānas, there is often reference to the form of an egg as a lingam. One could describe the principle of the world as a boundary, a curve that encircles the universe and forms the cosmic egg, "the golden egg

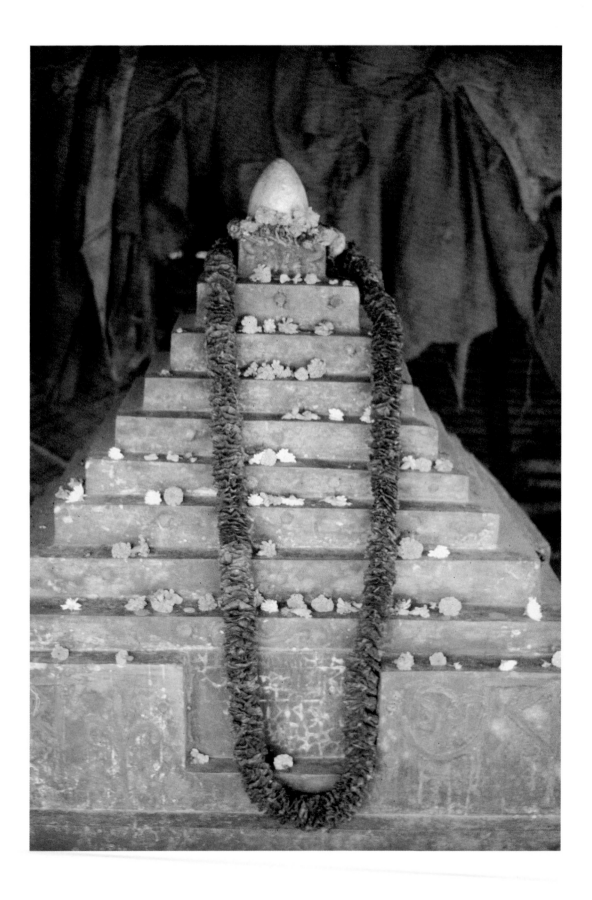

as resplendent as the sun" of Manu, the Great Legislator.

"According to Plutarch, the egg is the symbol of everything that remains sterile until the creator fertilizes them by the incubation of his vital spirit represented by a serpent. On medals coming from the colony of Tyr, an egg can be seen entwined by a serpent" (Payne Knight, *The Worship of Priapus*, p. 10).

The birth of the world from an egg, the image of totality, is a concept common to the Egyptians, Canaanites, Phoenicians, Greeks, Hindus, Celts, Chinese, Japanese, and Siberians. In Shinto, the primordial egg split into a light half (the sky) and a dense half (the earth). In Egyptian myth, a god wells up from the egg and makes order out of chaos, fashioning the embryos of the various forms of life. To the Incas, the supreme deity, Huiracocha, had the form of an egg.

We rediscover the myth of the cosmic egg in Africa among the Dogon and Bambara peoples of Mali. To the Koubs of the Congo, the white is the creative sperm and the yolk the feminine dampness that is the material of the creation.

The image of the egg as a symbol of resurrection, the periodical return of life, is perpetuated in the colored eggs of Easter. The eating of eggs was forbidden by Orphic regulations, whose goal was to free the soul of all its earthly attachments and all reincarnations.

◆

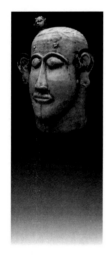

4

◆

INDIRECT REPRESENTATIONS OF THE PHALLUS

A phallic significance is often attributed to certain objects or animals, thus permitting the mention of the sex organ allegorically, according to a principle similar to those by which the pronunciation of the name of God is forbidden.

The phallus can thereby be evoked with the help of various symbols. Aside from the fish, the bird, and the serpent, the principle symbols are the bull, the horn, the moon, the foot, the thumb, the standing stone, the column, and the tree. It is often through the medium of such substitutes that the generational power continues to be worshiped in numerous religions. There is probably no religion in which a substratum of the phallic cult does not exist. In folklore, the most utilized symbol is probably the horn, as the bull is the animal form of the god.

During the period of prehistory dating from 6500 to 2000 B.C. in Western Europe, the male sex organ was identified by the plow, the axe, the dagger, the sword, semen, sperm, rain, the sun, serpents, fish, and birds.

On certain Greek vases are represented festivals in which large phalluses resembling fish are carried. . . . A relationship between the male sex organ and the fish was established very early ... and has become universal.... It is the same history for the bird. The winged phalluses of the ancient Greeks can be seen in the sanctuary of Delos ... these phallic birds, represented as geese or cocks, play an important role in European folk art, from which comes the word *cock* for the penis in English. Actually, it is a question of certain survivals of a ritual terminology that is reminiscent of certain Tantric rites. In regard to sperm offerings produced by masturbatory practices, the phallus is the fish. In initiation rites that include anal penetration, it is the bird (the bird is always the symbol of an esoteric significance). In fertility rites and sexual union it is always the bull (Philip Rawson, *Primitive Erotic Art*, pp. 21, 45, 53, and 71).

In popular Italian terminology the male sex organ, even today, is called *uccello* (bird) or *pesce* (fish).

In the Christian myth of the Nativity, the Holy Spirit is represented as a bird.

India: Phallic representations in a tapestry by the Assam tribe. Collection of Jacques Cloarec.

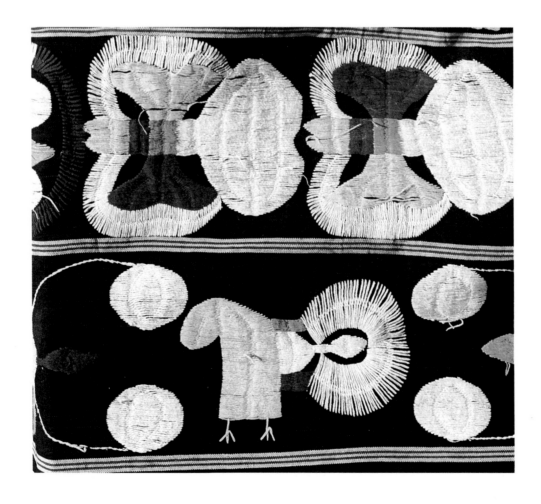

As the phallus was synonymous with power, the royal scepter originally took the form of one.

Until the nineteenth century in Italy, the character of Harlequin held a scepter from which dangled two testicles (Rawson, p. 20).

THE ARROW (BĀNA LINGAM)

The arrow, which evokes the creative organ that opens in order to fertilize, is the symbol of the number five because of the five arrows with which the god of love attacks the five senses. Therefore, the arrow is symbolically linked to the underlying principles of sensorial perception and to the five elements. In all symbolic orders, five is the number of Shiva. Inasmuch as the arrow is also the lingam, it is represented with five faces.

THE ALTAR FIRE

In sacrificial rites, fire, image of the Destroyer, is called its sign, its lingam. It is the light of Shiva *(shiva-jyotis)*. The altar represents the woman; the *yajña-kunda*, the hearth hollowed at the top of the altar,

Greece: Fish phallus carried in the Haloa Harvest Festival, 500 B.C. Athens. From the Staatliche Museen zu Berlin, Germany.

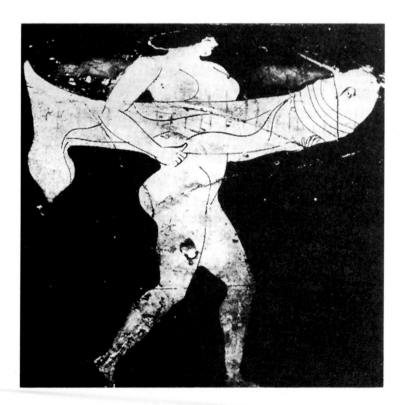

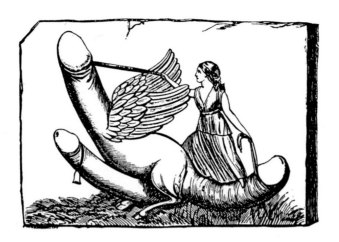

is the yoni. The ritual flame is obtained by the rotation of a pestle in a wooden bowl. "Fire, obtained by friction, is considered to be the progeny of a sexual union" (Mircea Eliade, *Histoire des croyances et des idées religieuses,* p. 437).

Italy: Bas-relief of phallic amulet, circa second century. Rome.

THE PLOW

The plow conjures up fertilization. The plowshare, like the virile member, penetrates the furrow opened by the plow in the female earth. Sītā, "born of the furrow," is the wife of the god Rāma in the Indian epic. The plow, which impregnates the field, evokes the union of man and woman, sky and earth. There is a linguistic family relationship between *lāngala,* the spade, and *lingam,* the phallus.

On ancient vases discovered in Abruzzi, the plowshare has the form of a phallus. A Greek vase in a museum in Florence depicts a phallus-shaped plow carried by ithyphallic men.

◆

Indirect Representations of the Phallus

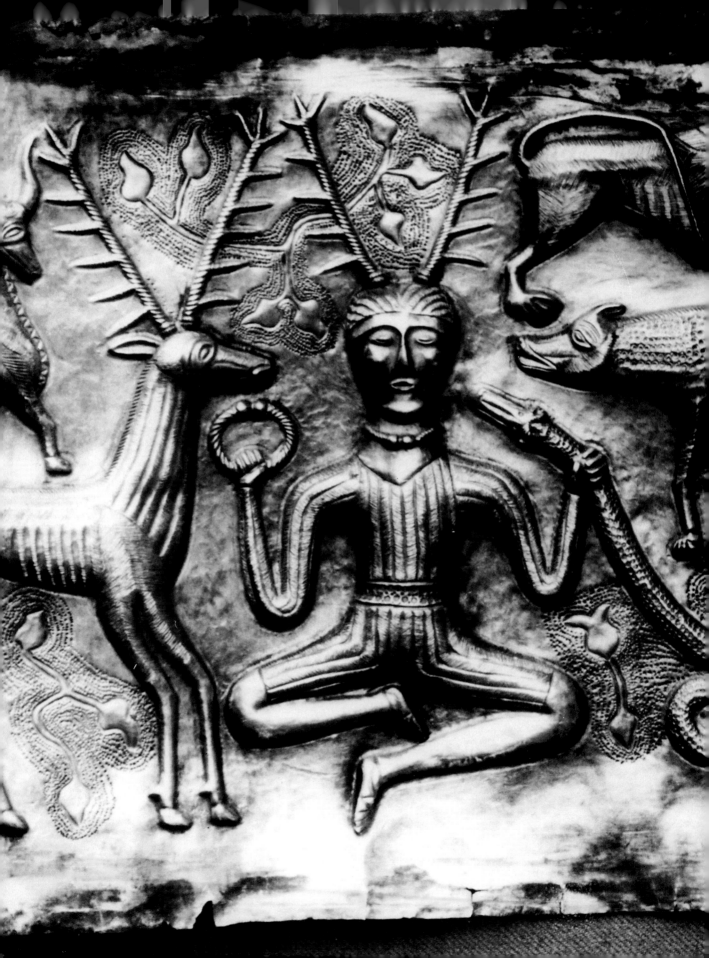

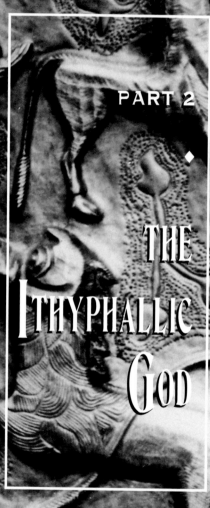

PART 2

◆

THE ITHYPHALLIC GOD

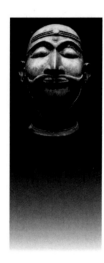

5

◆

THE LORD OF THE ANIMALS

The god whose emblem is the phallus first appears as a shepherd god, the friend of beasts, wandering in the forest with his penis erect and fascinating all creatures. The Hindu Purānas have preserved numerous descriptions of this strange and sacred character and of his adventures. This shepherd god who lives in the forest is to be found in all cultures, whether as Egypt's Min, Amon, Ra, Osiris, or even Pan, Priapus, or the god of the groves—Sylvanus. Faunus, the ancient god of Rome, the guardian of herds, vines, gardens, and shepherds, was assimilated into Pan.

Images of the ithyphallic horned god surrounded by animals can be found at Mohenjo Daro and Harappa (three thousand years before our own era), and they can be rediscovered as far as the famous Gundestrup cauldron in Denmark (circa 100 B.C.), where his image is practically identical with that at Mohenjo Daro.

The lord of the animals is, without any doubt, the descendant of the ancient mistress of the animals of Paleolithic times, whose characteristics, props, attributes, and legends are virtually the same as those of Pashupati, the Indian lord of the animals. This prodigious antiquity serves to explain how its trace can be found in all later civilizations.

"There was a tradition of lunar notation as early as the Aurignacian-Perigordian [32,000 B.C.], and ... a mythology that included a 'goddess' in storied relation to animals.... the 'goddess' with the horn is a fore-runner of later Neolithic, agricultural variants. She was the goddess who was called 'Mistress of the Animals,' had a lunar mythology, and had associated with her signs, symbols, and attributes, including the lunar crescent, the crescent horns of the bull, the fish, the angle-signs of water, the vulva, the naked breasts, the plant, flower, bird, tree, and snake. This later goddess was associated in story with a consort or mate who was ... the 'sun' to the goddess' 'moon'" (Alexander Marshack, *The Roots of Civilization*, p. 335–36).

It was under the name of Pan, god of the universe, that the cult of the god-phallus arrived in Greece, by way of Anatolia, about 500 B.C., *pan* meaning "all." He incarnates the whole of genetic energy, the totality of gods, the whole of life. Pan is the god of shepherds and flocks. His cult soon spilled over the borders of the Hellenic world. This god loves forests and springs. He is carefree and lazy. It is dangerous to disturb his sleep. Half man and half goat, bearded, horned, hairy, quick, hidden, a nimble runner, he lies in wait for nymphs and young boys, who are equally objects of his lust. His sexual hunger is insatiable, and he also indulges in masturbation.

He is, like Shiva, a musician and a dancer. He participates in the

Italy: Flute player sporting a phallus. Bronze. Museum of Rome.

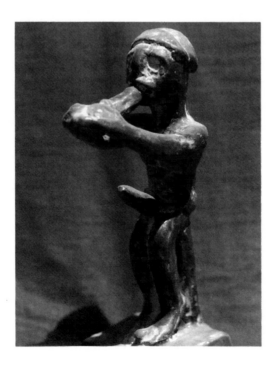

The Lord of the Animals

dances of the mountain nymphs. His attributes are the Pan flute and the flute of seven reeds. He carries a shepherd's staff, a crown, and branches of pine. He is part of the procession of Dionysus. He is the companion of Bacchus during the latter's expedition to India. According to a Homeric hymn, he is the son of Hermes and a nymph.

"Pan, with his enormous sexual organ, is the Priapus of Roman poets" (Payne Knight, *The Worship of Priapus*).

"Shiva travels in the forests and the jungles. He is called Pashupati, lord of the wild beasts" (*Shatapatha Brāhmana*, XII, 7.3.20).

Shiva's flock was composed of all living beings, including man. The only difference between animals, men, and gods is the role they play and their level in a continuous hierarchy. In all forms of existence, on various levels, the different aspects of the individual are present. There is no god without animality, no animal without humanity, no man without a portion of divinity.

"Dionysus was not a man; he was an animal and at the same time a god, thereby embodying the terminal points of the oppositions that man bears within himself" (Giorgio Colli, *La Sapienza Greca*, p. 15).

In every man can be distinguished three components called *pati*, *pashu*, and *pāsha*. Those in whom the element *pati* (master) dominates are the sages, kindred of the gods, who understand the rules of the divine game—creation—and participate therein. The majority of mankind in whom the animal element predominates are called *pashu* (livestock). An abstract element, *pāsha* (the bond or snare), expresses the unity and interdependence of all life forms. *Pāsha*, the snare, represents the group of laws that hold together the different elements of matter and the living being trapped in that creation.

No other morality exists outside of respect for the *pāsha*, the bond—that is, the interdependence of the animal and the divine within ourselves, the realization of the place we occupy in the whole of the divine opus, the affinities that bind us to the animal and plant species, and the responsibilities that those relationships entail. *Pāsha* could be defined as natural law, which is to say divine law. A type of behavior that is not founded on respect for nature and *pāsha*, the pact that joins together man and the divine, has nothing in common with true religion. Any other moral code is nothing but a social convention that is valueless on the universal level. True morality consists in conforming to those fundamental laws on which creation is founded. Everywhere that the influence of the cult of Shiva has extended, we

THE PHALLUS

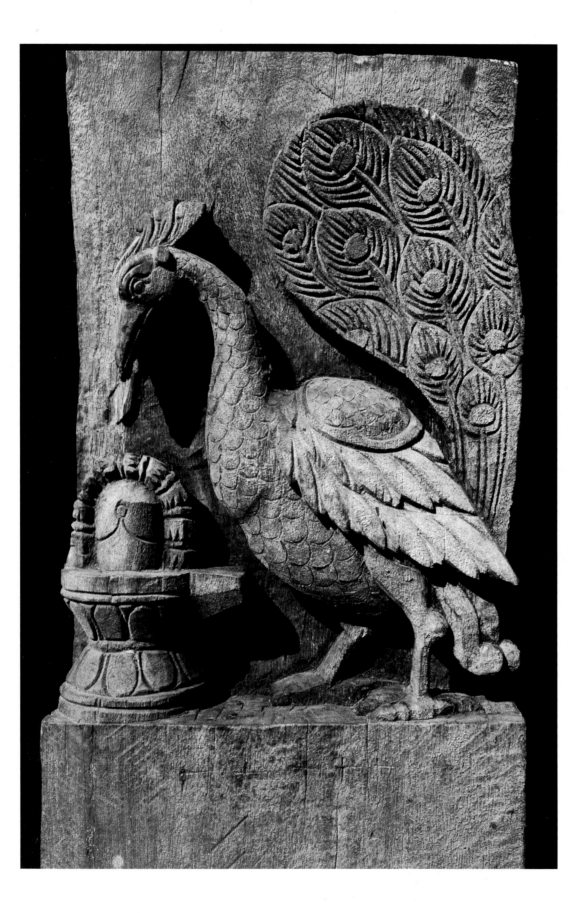

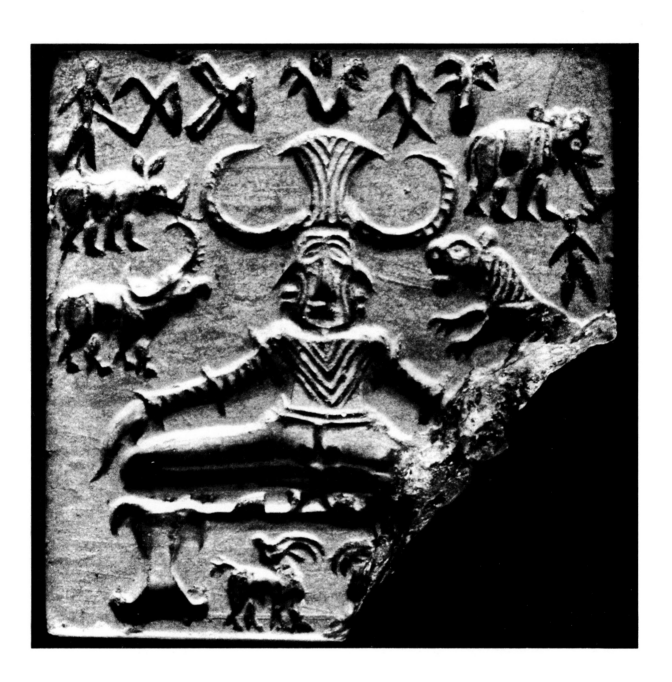

rediscover the importance of the animal and the plant kingdoms. This aspect of religious history seems to have often escaped the notice of modern specialists on the ancient world.

"One of the most obvious aspects of Greek culture—the role played by plants and animals in myth and legend—remains unexplained" (R. F. Willetts, *Cretan Cults and Festivals,* p. 60).

"Shiva looks at the gods and says to them: 'I am the lord of the animals.' The courageous Titans, the Asura, can be destroyed only if each of the gods and other beings assume their animal nature. The gods are hesitant to recognize their animal aspect. Shiva tells them: 'It is not degenerate to recognize one's animal' (the species in the animal kingdom corresponding to the principle that each god incarnates on the universal plane). Only those who practice the rites of the brothers to beasts, the *pashupāta,* can surpass their animal nature. It was thus that all the gods and the Titans recognized that they were the livestock of the Lord and that he was known under the name of Pashupati, the lord of the animals" (*Shiva Purāna, Rudra Samhitā,* 5.9.13–21).

To watch over the beasts and plants as well as men, Shiva created the *vidyeshvara* (masters of knowledge), who appeared as forest spirits, satyrs, nymphs, fairies, and guardian angels. These are creation's guardian spirits. Pashupati is the chief of these spirits, and through them manifests in every aspect of the natural world. Shiva dwells in the mountains and the forests; there his mysterious presence is felt, and it is there, within caverns or isolated locales, that shrines are built to him and offerings brought.

Very close to Shiva in symbolism and legend, Dionysus is the god of vegetation, vines, wine, fruits, and seasonal renewal. As principle and master of animal and human fertility, he is embodied in the form of the bull, the serpent, and the lion, who appear often in his legends and his cult. He is called Phallen or Phallenos.

By an interesting reversal occurring in mythical narratives, it is Dionysus who conquers India, teaching viniculture, establishing laws, and founding cities. In fact, the original habitat of the grape vine is India—the only region where it is naturally found in the wild.

The procession of the phallus plays an important role in his festivals. In the house of the Mysteries at Pompeii, we can see that the unveiling of the phallus was a part of Dionysian initiation rites.

"The sinuous serpent winding round the caduceus is once more in accordance with Celtic tradition. Again the horned god appears as a

OPPOSITE
India: Pashupati, lord of animals. Seal of Mohenjo Daro, circa 2500 B.C. With permission of the National Museum of New Delhi.

The Lord of the Animals

51

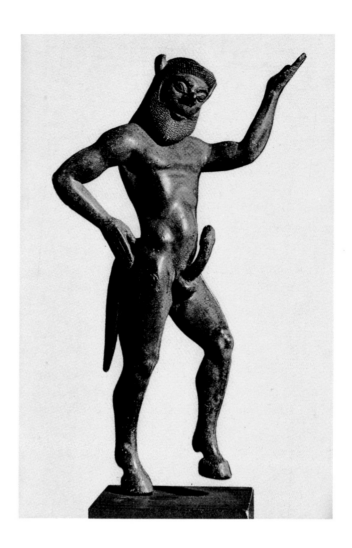

kind of native Silvanus, god of the woods, naked and without attribute
apart from his huge penis. In north Britain another type of naked phallic god is figured, but without the horns, therefore presumably of the
Cerne giant type, bearing arms or without attribute. A deity of similar
type, fierce and aggressively phallic, comes from Maastricht, Holland.
… The combination of horned beasts, ithyphallic men and other symbols, together with the close association of a spring and probably a
pool, indicate an ancient Caucasian fertility rite, somewhere between
1000 and 600 B.C." (Anne Ross, in *Primitive Erotic Art*, pp. 84–85).

The character of Shiva in his aspect of animal charmer and guardian
has often been transferred to later divinities such as Gopāla-Krishna,
Pan, Orpheus, and even Jesus, the Good Shepherd.

"All the deities are called *pashupāta* (brothers of the beasts), because they form part of Pashupati's flock. All who consider the lord of

the animals as their deity become beast brothers" (*Linga Purāna*, 80.56–57). They are then integrated into the flock of the god and capable of receiving his teachings.

"Shiva says: the very holy *pashupāta* yoga, the yoga of the beast brothers (by which the unity of all living beings can be realized) and the Sāmkhya cosmology (which explains the structure of the world), have been taught by me.... Knowing that the things of this world are ephemeral, it is necessary to continually practice the yoga of the animal lord" (*Linga Purāna*, 34.11–23).

THE GOD OF VEGETATION AND FERTILITY

In the Mediterranean tradition, the god Fascinus, who germinates plants and renders sterile women fertile, is personified by the phallus.

Priapus is the god of gardens and generation.

"During the course of certain Athenian festivals, women planted male sex organs as if they were sowing seed to ensure the fertility of the fields" (John Boardman and Eugenio La Rocca, *Eros en Grecia*, p. 40).

The modern concept of ecology can be seen as a tentative return to a true morality, even though it is often anthropocentric. It is not solely a question of preserving nature for man's use but rather of rediscovering man's proper role within nature, as a cooperative agent in the work of the gods. A religion that does not respect the indivisible whole of creation and that is not fundamentally ecological is nothing but a deception, an excuse for human depredations that in no case can proclaim any divine origins. Man is only one element of a group, and it is the entire group that is the work of God.

At times the phallic image has a fertilizing power. Daphne was born from a phallic column. Jeremiah invoked those who spoke to the stone: "You have fathered me" (Jeremiah 2:27).

According to Prometheus' history of Italy in the Etruscan language cited by Plutarch, a phallus appeared in the chimney of the king of Albe. He ordered his daughter to couple with this phallus, but she refused and sent her servant instead. From the servant were born Romulus and Remus, who were abandoned in the forest and suckled by a wolf.

The women of Veliae, in a prenuptial rite, had to couple with a phallus. This custom, also widespread among the Romans and described by

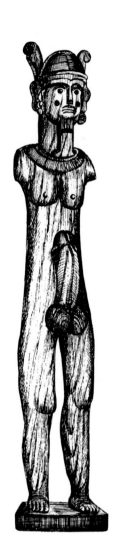

Indonesia: Wood sculpture representing an ithyphallic fertility god.

early Christian writers such as Lactance and Arnobus, is represented on a bas-relief in the secret museum of Pompei. The fiancee offered her virginity to the god in order to win his favors and to avoid sterility.

Even today, the young girls of Nepal have their hymens broken by means of a phallus-shaped fruit in a rite that grants to the god a sort of "droit du seigneur."

In various cultures where the rites of phallus worship have officially disappeared, numerous phallic images can be found whose presence is regarded as essential to insure the fertility of women and fields alike. This is the case in all of eastern Africa, in particular among the Yoruba. One often comes across those phallus-shaped altars that insure the fertility of the earth and to which are made offerings of sperm at the onset of the sowing season.

Analogous rites and images have existed until very recent times in the entire area of Oceania. Numerous images of an ithyphallic god are gathered in the museums of California.

Further on in this work we will investigate the fertilizing role of Santo Membro in medieval Europe, a role that has survived to the present day in central Italy.

"The belief in the fertilizing virtues of menhirs was still shared by European peasantry at the beginning of the century. In France, young women who desired to have children were in the habit of sliding down these stones or creating a similar friction by sitting atop the monoliths or rubbing their bellies against them" (Mircea Eliade, *Histoire des croyances et des idées religieuse*, 1.130).

THE SPIRIT OF THE FORESTS, THE LEWD AND NAKED GOD

"The gods and the prophets have been created naked. Every human being is created nude" (*Linga Purāna*, 1.34.13).

Nudity represents a return to the primordial state. The identification of man and god with nature implies nudity. David danced naked in front of the ark (2 Samuel 6:14). The true man is nude; it is the hypocritical and pharisaic religion of the cities that demands clothing. Shiva is naked, "clothed in space." The sage and the Shaivite monk wander the world naked and without attachments. Nudity is synonymous with liberty, virtue, truth, and holiness. The ancient atheist religion of India, Jainism, the rival of Shaivism in other regards, made similar demands of its faithful that they be naked. The Greek world was very fa-

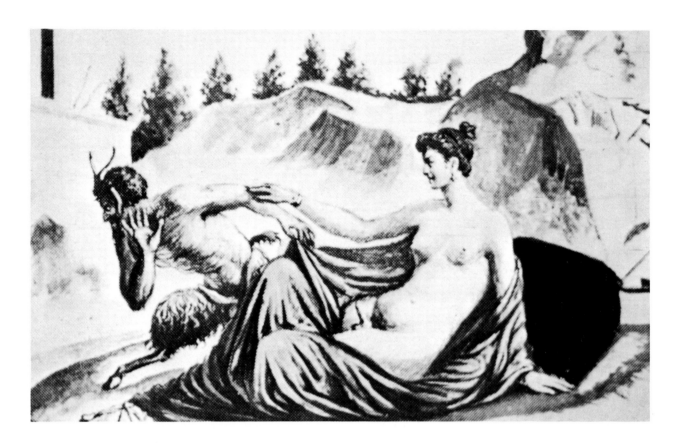

miliar with its gymnosophists, naked ascetics who came from India, and the soldiers of Alexander who wished to follow the teachings of Indian philosophers had to disrobe. Nudity has a sacred and magic value. "To sow your seed go naked, strip to plow and strip to reap, if you would harvest all Demeter's yield in season. Thus each crop will come in turn" (Hesiod, *Works and Days*, p. 390–95).

Ritual nudity is well known and widespread in ancient religions. Shinto priests purify themselves in nakedness, and it was in nakedness that Hebrew priests penetrated the Holy of Holies to signify their lack of ornamentation at the approach of the divine mystery. There are countless examples in Celtic literature where masculine nudity is closely connected with the warrior's trance. Celtic warriors went into combat naked. In the Irish mythological tale *The Destruction of Da Derga's Hostel,* the bird-father of the king says to him: "A man stark-naked, who shall go at the end of the night along one of the roads of Tara, having a sling and a stone, he shall be king" (Anne Ross, in *Primitive Erotic Art,* p. 81).

Dionysus himself is also represented as a long-haired nude when he is not clothed in a saffron-colored monk's robe.

Italy: Fresco reproduction of Hermaphrodite and the god Pan, early nineteenth century. Pompeii. From the private collection of Emde Boas. Photograph from Rufus Camphausen's Encyclopedia of Erotic Wisdom *(Inner Traditions).*

The Lord of the Animals

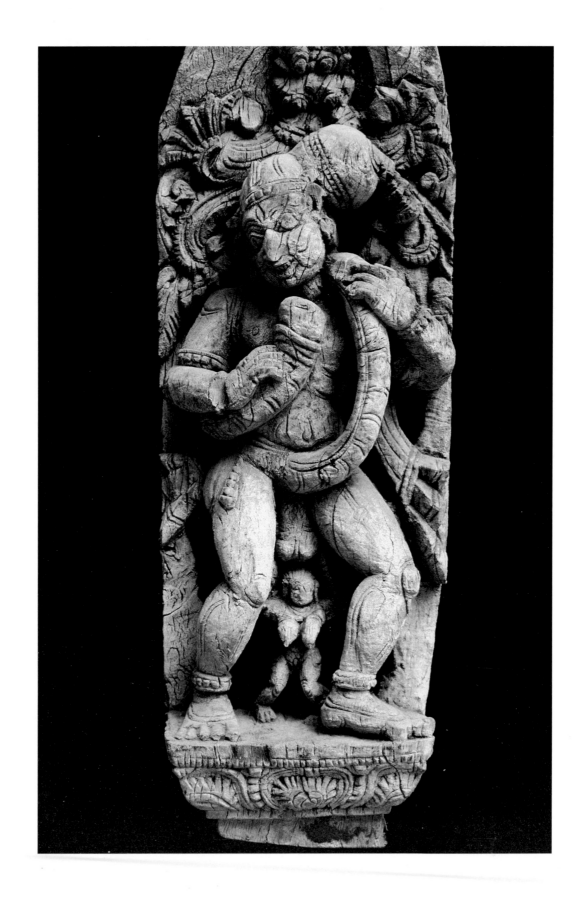

The legends of the Purānas depict Shiva as a lewd adolescent who roams naked in the forest, charming the women of the prideful ascetics who wish to conquer heaven by the force of their will. Shiva humiliates the ascetics, seduces their wives, and through spilling his semen here and there causes the earthly appearance of precious stones and sacred sites.

According to the *Shiva Purāna* (*Kothi Rudra Samhitā*, chapter 12): "There existed a large cedar forest called Dāruvana. A large number of hermit worshipers of Shiva lived there, ceaselessly meditating on the creator of the world. Three times a day they performed ritual prayers to their lord and sang hymns to his glory. One day while the hermits were off in the forest seeking the sacred herbs they used in their rites, Shiva, to test their faith, embodied himself in a strange form. He appeared resplendent and totally naked. His body was coated in ashes with no other ornamentation. He stood there with his penis in his hand and started making an exhibition of himself with obscene acts. Shiva had come to this place to display the benevolence he felt toward his faithful who were the inhabitants of this forest.

"The lord had the appearance of a man of low estate. In his hand a flaming torch shook. His eyes were red and brown. Sometimes he would laugh uproariously; sometimes he would sing in an astonishing manner. Sometimes he danced lasciviously; sometimes he cried out. He wandered around the hermitages like a beggar.... Despite his dark-colored skin, he was of a surprising beauty. He laughed and sang, winking at the women in such a way that they were utterly captivated. He, who had vanquished the god of love, inspired desire by his beauty alone. Despite his strange appearance and his tanned skin, the most chaste women were attracted to him" (*Linga Purāna*, 1.29.7, 10, 12, and 1.31.28–32).

"The wives of the hermits were frightened at first sight. Despite their surprise, many felt drawn to the god and approached him. Some sought to embrace him, others to seize hold of his hands. They began to fight among themselves for the privilege of touching him" (*Shiva Purāna, Kothi Rudra Samhitā*, 12.9).

"At a smile on his lips, those women before their huts and those living in the treetops dropped their work. They tore off their clothes and let their hair down. Some even rolled in the dirt. They clutched at one another and, blocking the god's path, made lewd gestures to him in the absence of their husbands. The lord said nothing to them, neither good

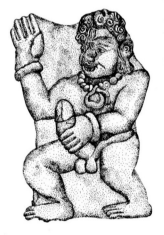

ABOVE
India: Mukteshvara Temple, Bhuvaneshvar. Ithyphallic dwarf, twelfth century.
OPPOSITE
India: Shiva as youth with elongated phallus. Photograph by Lance Dane.

The Lord of the Animals

nor evil" (*Linga Purāna,* 1.29.7—9). Here can be seen another version of the conduct of the maenads, and the name given to Dionysus: *Gynaimanes* (he who drives women mad).

"It is at this moment that the sages returned. Seeing this naked man giving free rein to obscene acts, they were scandalized and entered in a rage. Deceived by Shiva's power of illusion and blinded by their prejudice, they cried out: 'What's going on here? What is the meaning of this? Say, who is this? Say, who is this?' But the naked figure made no response to their queries" (*Shiva Purāna, Kothi Rudra Samhitā,* 12.14).

"The priests and sages gave utterance to words of indignation, but the power of their virtues was ineffective against Shiva, in the same way that the glow of the stars can do nothing against the light of the sun" (*Linga Purāna,* 1.29.9, 24).

"The sages cried out: 'This Shiva who carries a trident has an ill-omened body. Has he no shame? He has no dwelling nor any known ancestors. He is naked and poorly formed. He lives in the company of bad and evil spirits. . . . If he had any money he wouldn't be running around naked. He goes about on a bull; he has no other carriage. His caste is unknown; he is neither learned nor wise. He has none in his retinue but evil spirits. He is up to his neck in poison. Compare your necklaces to the garland of skulls he wears, your cosmetics to the ashes from funeral pyres with which he covers his body'" (*Shiva Purāna, Rudra Samhitā,* 24.45—47 and 27.36).

"When the naked figure didn't respond, the hermits hurled even greater imprecations against the terrible man-god: 'You comport yourself in an indecent manner. You have violated the rules of the Veda. May your penis fall to the ground!' The moment these words were uttered, the penis of the divine envoy, who was none other than Shiva of the splendid body, fell to the ground. But it burned everything in its path. Everywhere it went, everything caught fire and was burnt. It descended into the depths of the infernos; it rose into the very heavens; it ravaged the entire earth. No spot remained unpenetrated by it. All worlds and beings were in great distress. The hermits were terrified. No longer could either gods or wise men experience any peace or joy. Finally Shiva vanished.

"The gods and the hermits who hadn't known enough to recognize him were full of consternation. They gathered together and went to the maker of the world, the god Brahmā, to implore him for protec-

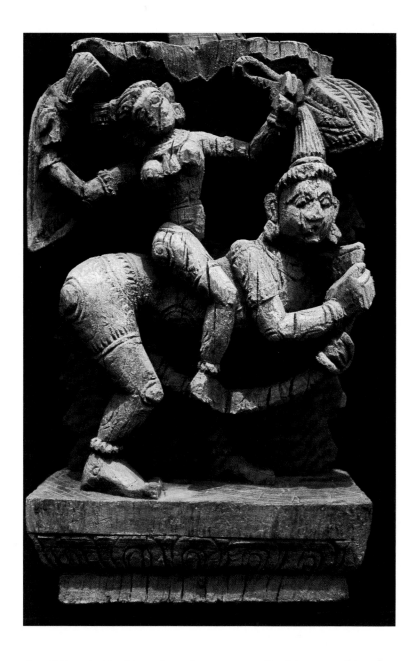

India: Shiva mounted by female who uses his elongated phallus as a bridle. Photograph by Lance Dane.

tion. After singing his praises, they recounted to him everything that had occurred. Brahmā said to them: 'How stupid you are! In one moment you have destroyed all the credits you acquired by your practice of abstinence. That man with the erect penis that you have seen—impotents that you are—is the Supreme Lord in person' " (*Linga Purāna*, 1.29.9–25).

" 'How is it possible that you, who are wise, could commit such errors? How can you condemn the poor ignoramus for his faults when you behave just like him? Who then could expect to recover their

The Lord of the Animals

serenity after having offended Shiva so gravely? When someone refuses to honor an unforeseen guest who appears at his door at mealtime, all credit earned by one's practice of abstinence is carried away by the visitor, who leaves in return the weight of all his misdeeds. What can happen when that visitor is Shiva himself? As long as the sex organ of the god remains unstabilized, nothing good can occur in any of the three worlds. Such is the truth.

" 'To calm his rage, you must erect a stone phallus and water this divine sex organ with holy water. You must construct a pedestal for it in the form of a vagina and an arrow [symbol of the goddess] and install it with prayers, offerings, acts of self-abasement, hymns, and songs accompanied by musical instruments. Then you must call forth the god by saying: "You are the source of the universe, the origin of the universe. You are present in all that exists. O Benevolent One! Calm down and protect the world." ' The sages then piously approached Shiva, who said to them: 'The world will not find peace until my penis has found a receptacle. No other than the Lady of the mountain can lay hold of my penis. If she grasps it, it will calm down immediately' " (*Shiva Purāna, Kothi Rudra Samhitā*, 12.22–46).

CASTRATION

The emasculation of the masculine sky related by Hesiod is tied to the same symbolism. According to the *Theogony* (188 ff.), Aphrodite was born from the sex organ of Ouranos, which had been thrown into the sea and surrounded by a white foam that evoked the semen of the emasculated heavens. *Aphrodite* means "foam."

Italy: Sculpture of severed phallus, first century. Rome. Collection of Jacques Cloarec.

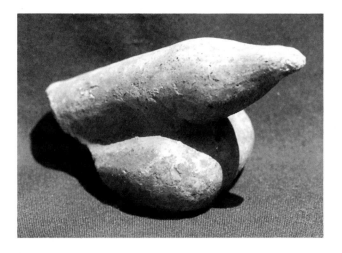

"The castration of Ouranos puts an end to a period of uninterrupted procreation, evoking the tendency of the gods to withdraw after having completed their cosmogonical work. In Hurrute and Hittite theogony, Kumarbi, the father of the gods, pursued Anu, and seizing him by the feet, flung him to the ground after having bitten off his penis. A fraction of Anu's virility penetrated his body, and he became pregnant with three gods" (Mircea Eliade, *Histoire des croyances et des idées religieuses,* pp. 150 and 159).

In Egypt, the broken and truncated body of the agrarian deity Osiris, murdered by his brother Seth and thrown into the Nile, was reassembled anew by Isis, except for his penis, which had been eaten by a fish.

In Greece, the young and beautiful Phrygian shepherd Attis, the lover of Rhea, was mutilated during a burst of insanity. His faithful practiced orgiastic celebrations and, in an extreme ritual, cut off and deposited their virile organs on the altars of Attis and Rhea. A similar practice exists as well in India, among the impassioned worshipers of the goddess Kālī.

◆

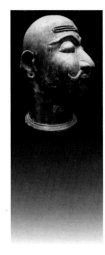

6

♦

THE GUARDIAN GOD

HERMES

The phallus serves as protection against the evil eye, danger and misfortune.

"Every street corner in Athens had its cippus dedicated to Hermes, a square pilaster topped with the god's head and on which were sculpted genital organs in erection, which bypassers would touch for luck, because all luck is a gift from Hermes" (John Boardman and Eugenio La Rocca, *Eros en Grecia,* p. 40).

"In the countrysides there were columns erected at every crossroads to protect travelers from phantoms and unfortunate encounters. The Hermaic pillars were originally utilized as funerary symbols, but their multiplication along country, then city, roads, at crossroads, in town squares, and finally in houses is certainly due to the protective virtues they were assumed to possess. Like the rustic images of Priapus, they averted the evil eye, and popular piety attributed to them a beneficial power. While never reaching the importance of Dionysus in the Greek area, Hermes, in the form of a pillar with genitalia, has largely profited from the cult of the phallus favored by the Dionsysian ritual" (Jean Mercadé, *Eros Kalos,* p. 89).

The name of Hermes derives from Hermaï—the cairn, or heap of

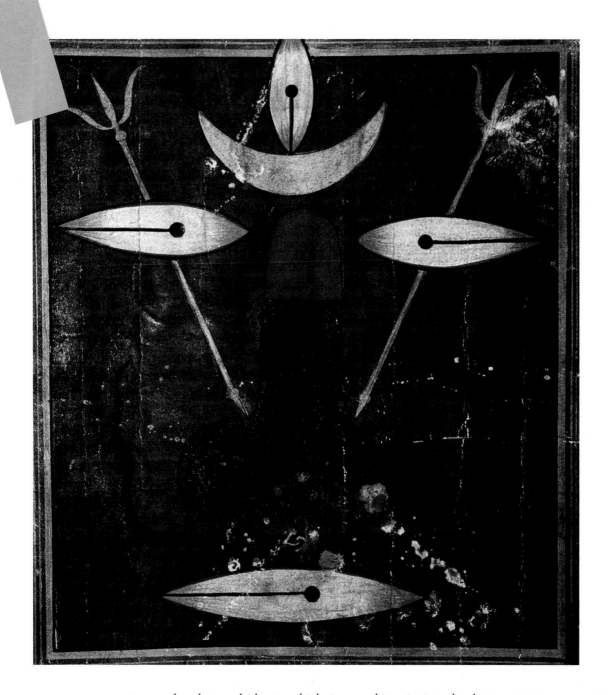

stones, placed at roadsides, to which since prehistoric times has been attributed both a protective and a fertilizing presence. Transformed into columns and crowned with a head, the stones became the image of the god that bore their name (see p. 10). The Apollo cult derived in equal measure from these stone piles, which were always distinctive signs of the sun god as well.

Legend places the birth of Hermes in a cavern on Mount Cyllene, and the product of the rape by Zeus of Maïa, the goddess Earth. His

India: Tantric phallic painting. Photograph by Lance Dane.

The Guardian God

mother deposited him in a ritually consecrated willow basket. The master of animals, Hermes is the guardian of shepherds, flocks, and travelers delayed on the roads. He is cunning and deceitful, like Skanda, the son of Shiva, the god of thieves and looters. A treatise on the art of theft, the *Sanmukha Kalpa*, is attributed to Skanda. Barely out of the womb, Hermes stole Apollo's cattle. He stretched one of their hides on a tortoise shell and added a pair of horns, from which he then strung cords of gut, creating the first lyre. With the mysterious power of his music, he established the bond that ties together art and the mysteries. Presiding over the divinatory arts, he possessed a magic wand, the caduceus, and a cap that conferred invisibility upon its wearer. The equivalent of the Celtic Lug and the Egyptian Thot, he is the master of the initiate. He watches over the civilizing Hero, patron of the occult sciences, through the intermediary of the initiatory scenario, the sacrality of the sexual undertaking, vegetal fertility and nourishment. In the Eleusinian ritual, linked to an agrarian mysticism, the tray of offerings contained a phallus and a serpent or even cakes shaped like phalluses.

Hermes was also the inventor of fire, which was created by the friction of the male pestle in the feminine mortar. During spring sowing festivals, a large phallus representing Hermes was promenaded across the city, and orgiastic dances took place around the god's columns.

On the eve of the 415 B.C. expedition to Sicily, Alcibiades provoked the consternation of the city when he mutilated the Hermes columns in the public square of Athens in an act of defiance.

PRIAPUS

The name Priapus seems to be a derivative of the word *briapnos* (noisy) and would therefore be a translation of the Indian Rudra, the Howler.

Priapus, born as the result of an adventure between Dionysus and Aphrodite, was an ugly child possessing enormous genitals. He was reputedly a native of Lampsachus in Mysia. His cult spread to the Aegean islands and thence to Rome, where it blended into those of Pan and even more specifically into that cult of the ancient Etruscan phallic deity called Mutinus-Tutinus or Tutinus-Mutinus (from *muto*, the virile member).

As a gardening god, Priapus carries a pruning knife. He is responsible for the safeguarding of vineyards and orchards. He is represented under an ithyphallic form because that attribute deflects any evil spell that could cause harm to the crops. Very highly regarded by the people of Rome, he was represented there as Hermes, by a cippus topped with a head and adorned with an erect phallus.

The Priapus of Verona carries a basket full of phalluses, along with a serpent biting his penis.

In Rome the image of Priapus, painted with cinnabar or vermilion, was placed in entranceways for protection. The phallus bestowed good luck while dispelling danger and driving away the forces seeking to do evil. It played an important role in initiation rites. "In Egypt as well as in the Greco-Roman world the powerful temples attributed to the phallus the power of paralyzing or dispelling dark and demonic forces" (Julius Evola, *Le Yoga tantrique*, p. 112). In Rome, according to Macrobus, a phallus of great size was suspended upon the chariots of victorious generals because of the maxim *fortuna gloriae carnifex,* success destroys luck. Only the presence of the Fascinus permitted one to confront this dreadful test of success.

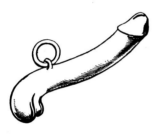 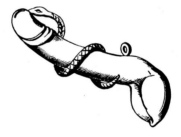

Phallic amulets.

"The phallus possesses a magical power that is particularly effective against the evil eye. . . . This is why one finds so many phallic amulets and so many sex organs carved on the walls of houses, in Greek Delos, just as in Pompei" (John Boardman and Eugenio La Rocca, *Éros en Grecia*, p. 42).

"Those who steadfastly worship the Great God under the form of the phallus are freed from fear and the cycle of birth and death" (*Linga Purāna*, 2.6.40). In India, the image of the lingam and the representations of sexual couplings protect house and temple against lightning and other calamities.

"Another type of early portrayal of the human figure, the sexual potency and fertility associations of which cannot be in question, is found

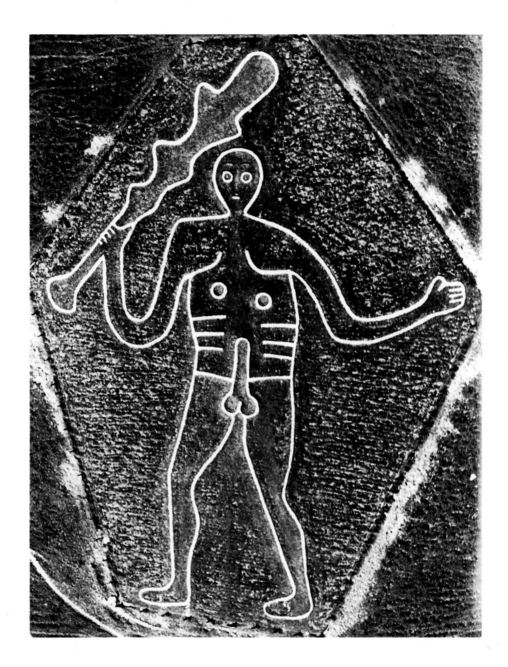

British Isles: Drawing on the earth of Cerne Abbas Giant, circa first century B.C. Dorset.

widely in Europe. . . . In general, they consist of representations of emphatically phallic men engaged in some activity such as hunting, fighting, sorcery or ball-games. . . . Somewhat later in date, belonging perhaps to the early Romano-British period, is the famous chalk-cut figure on the hill above Cerne Abbas, Dorset. Known as the Cerne Abbas giant, this British 'Hercules' with his all-conquering club, like that of the great Irish god Dagda, and his huge penis and testicles, has survived through the centuries, dominating the surrounding countryside, defying the Church, and remaining down to the present day a powerful fertility symbol. Young couples about to be married still resort to him, and it was believed in the district that to have sexual intercourse within the hollow of the vast phallus could only have beneficial results" (Anne Ross, in *Primitive Erotic Art*, pp. 81–82).

"There are numerous references and hints in European literature to the fact that not only art-made objects but actual human genitals were felt to have a magical power, especially in averting all kinds of misfortunes" (Philip Rawson, *Primitive Erotic Art*, p. 76).

In the popular conception that still thrives today in the countries of the Mediterranean, men touch their sex to avert the evil eye and make the evocative gesture of the *mano impudica* to invoke luck. Realistic and symbolic emblems of the male sex organ have often been planted in their fields by agrarian peoples. In southern Italy, phallic markers serving as boundaries have survived into the present day. Some of these were stone blocks from which emerged a phallus, sometimes accompanied with a human head as well. They were called Priapus, Hermes, Liber, Tutinus, or Mutinus (Rawson, pp. 52 and 82).

The Shaivites wear a small phallus at their throats, as did the ancient Romans. Numerous examples of this can be seen at Pompeii. In India a stone lingam is worshiped in every household, and large wooden phal-

Nepal: Ek Mukh lingam of Shiva. Kathmandu. Photograph by Kevin Bubriski.

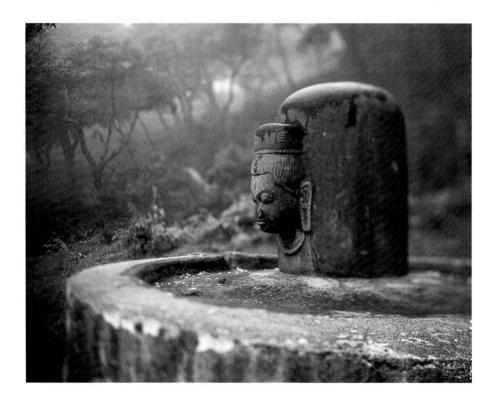

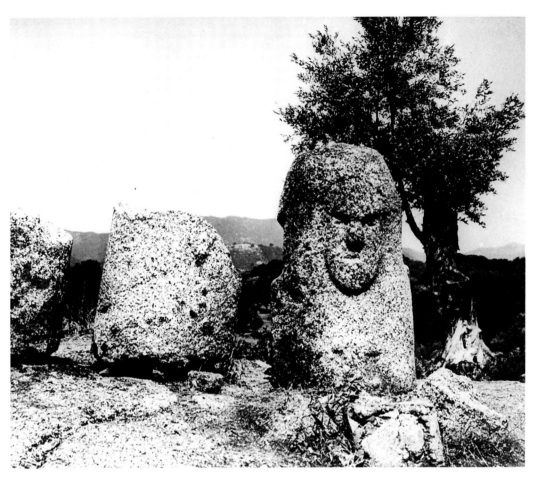

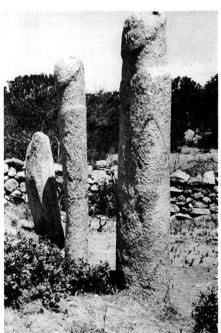

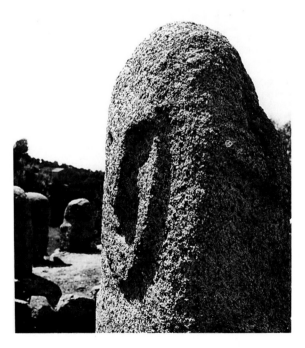

luses are carried in holy processions. Herodotus mentions the carrying of phallic emblems in the processions of Dionysus and Osiris. "The figures with disproportionately large phalluses that the Egyptians carried in procession during the festival of Osiris were stored in the Temple of Hieropolis, in Syria" (J.-A. Dulaure, *Des Divinités génératrices et du culte du phallus*, p. 82).

The god Priapus ruled over the phallophorias of each and every god. Men and women alike participated in erotic songs and orgies. In the agrarian cycles of Athens, cakes were made in the forms of phalluses or of serpents, the pieces of which were blended in with seeds. In Rome, "an ass was sacrificed to Priapus and offerings of flowers, fruits, milk, and honey were made to him" (Dulaire, op. cit., p. 83).

"Until very recently phallic cakes were baked by German, French and Italian peasants at Easter to be carried in procession to the church." "At Trani, by Naples, a huge wooden phallic image called Il Santo Membro was carried in procession annually until the eighteenth century" (Philip Rawson, *Primitive Erotic Art*, pp. 53; 75).

"The habit of placing a phallus on the walls of buildings, a practice that came from the Romans, still existed in the Middle Ages, and the edifices most specifically placed under the influence of this symbol were churches, where they served as protection against all kinds of enchantment, in which the population of that time lived constantly in fear. They protected not only the place they adorned and those who frequented it, but also those who looked on it from afar with faith. They were usually placed at doorways, like that of the cathedral of Toulouse and several other churches in Bordeaux and elsewhere in France. But, during the Revolution, they were destroyed by an ignorant populace who saw in them a sign of the clergy's depravity" (Payne Knight, *The Worship of Priapus*, p. 114). A wooden phallus can still be seen today in the basilica of St. Bertrand of Comminges.

THE GOD OF THE HUMBLE

Shiva, god of the pre-Aryan peoples of India, remained their preferred deity, even after their enslavement and degradation to the stature of artisan castes in the world dominated by their invaders. The *Hymn of the One Hundred Rudra* of the *Vājaseneya Samhitā* (*Yajur Veda*, 16.1) invokes him as the patron of craftsmen, cart drivers, carpenters, blacksmiths, potters, hunters, water bearers, and woodsmen.

The Guardian God

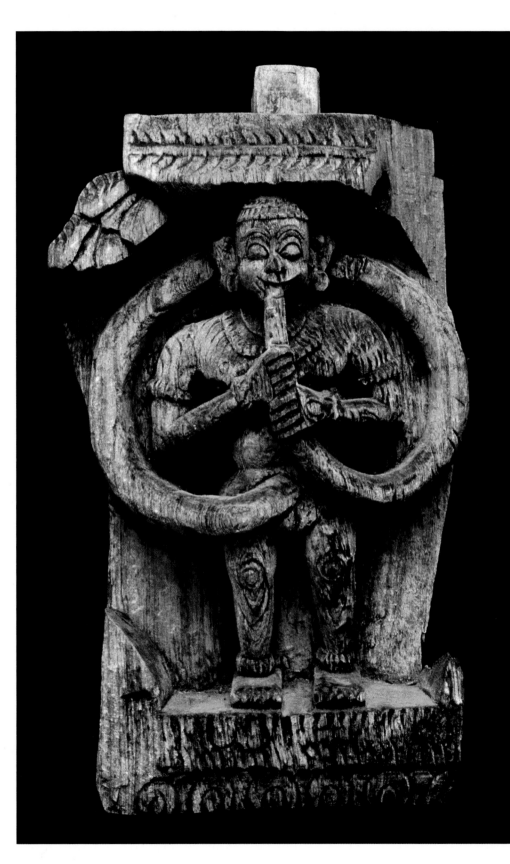

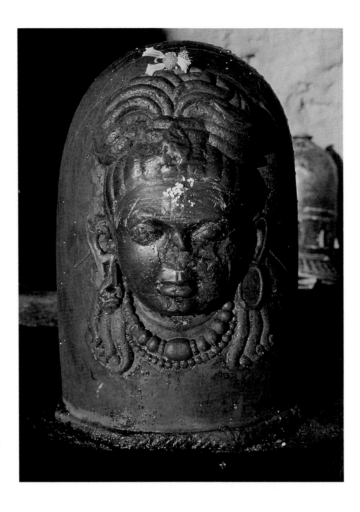

He is the god of soldiers, mercenaries, and the intrepid chariot driver. Shiva is also the god of the *vrātya*, the ascetic beggars and wanderers (P. Banerjee, *Early Indian Religions*, p. 41).

"In Shaivism, transcendence in relation to the norms of everyday life is translated on the popular plane by the fact that Shiva, among others, is represented as the god or "patron" of those who do not lead a normal life and even those who are outlaws" (Julius Evola, *Le Yoga tantrique*, p. 91).

Shiva was the god of the humble; his teachings were addressed to all mankind. Brahmanic texts reproach him for having taught the lower classes the secrets of the myths, the rituals, and the highest levels of knowledge and for having opened the path of initiation to them. Phallic rites are essentially folk rites. The *Shatapatha Brāhmana* (5.3.2) mentions the *shūdra*, the artisans, as participants in sacrifices to Shiva and to *soma*, the sacred liquor absorbed as the sperm of the god. Even

The Guardian God

today, in the most important Shaivite shrines, the service is practiced alternately by Aryan brahman priests and *shūdra* worker-priests. A non-Aryan priesthood has therefore survived throughout the centuries, despite four thousand years of Aryan domination. "In the mahratta regions, where the Shaivites predominate, brahmans do not officiate in the temples. That function is reserved to a special caste, called *gurava*, which is of *shūdra* origin, not Aryan" (P. Banerjee, *Early Indian Religion,* p. 41). The traditions of these non-Aryan priests are poorly known in a Hindu world dominated by high castes that if not Aryan are totally Aryanized. No modern study concerning them exists.

◆

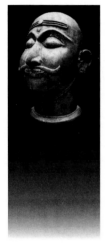

7

◆

The Animal and Plant Forms of the God

THE BULL

The cult of the phallus, since its inception, has been associated with that of the bull, which is considered the vehicle of the ithyphallic god and its alter ego in the animal kingdom. Every place that witnessed the spread of the cult also contains evidence of bulls and horns considered as symbols of power, virile potency being synonymous with sexual and divine power.

In Greece and Rome, the goat has at times taken the place of the bull, but in India, the bull remains the sacred animal and its image can be found before the entrance of every shrine where the lingam is worshiped. The devotees touch the animals' testicles before entering the temple, where they venerate the divine phallus with flowers, incense, and offerings.

On Greek medals, the auroch, or wild bull, is represented butting against the cosmic egg and lifting it with his horns. In the Orphic hymns the god is called *tauromorphos*.

"Evil-working genies, born of Vishnu's union with the daughters of the Titans, sowed terror throughout heaven and earth. Shiva took the form of a bull and exterminated them" (*Shiva Purāna, Shata Rudra*

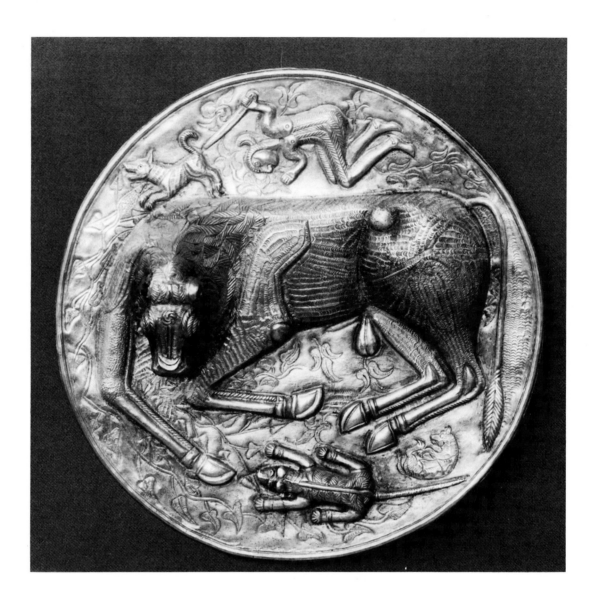

Bronze amulet of bull. National Museum of Copenhagen.

Samhitā, chap. 23). In times of danger, the Canaanite god, Baal, would also regain his primal form of the cosmic bull.

The bull is the vehicle of Shiva. The bull is Shiva. It is the embodiment in the animal kingdom of the principle represented by the ithyphallic god. Apis, the ox, is identified with the castrated Osiris. The bull is the ancient Cretan god worshiped since the time of greatest antiquity. "Son of the earth . . . symbol of the active principle producing semen, the bull was a sacred symbol in all societies that domesticated cattle" (Paolo Santarcangeli, *Il Libro dei Labirinti*, p. 234). The bull is associated with the very idea of the supreme and great divinity. According to Jean-Clarence Lambert (*Labrynthes et dédales du monde*,

p. 10), the Sanskrit word *go* (bull) is one of the etymological roots of the word that signifies "god," giving us the Scandinavian Gud, the German Gott, and the English God. In the Anatolia of 7000 B.C., as in Minoan Crete, the male god has the form of a bull or is associated with one. In the same era indicated by the Purānas as that which saw the diffusion of Shaivism (circa 7000 B.C.), one finds in Anatolia, at Çatal Hüyük, the first representations of God as a young boy or adolescent, and even as a bearded man, mounted on his sacred animal, the bull. The skulls of bulls were hung on the walls.

The ithyphallic god can be seen on an image of Shiva coming from Mohenjo Daro (2000 B.C.), seated in a yoga position. He is wearing a crown of bulls' horns. Several horned masks and representations of humpbacked bulls, as well as a unicorn bull, can be found there also. Ctesias and Aristotle both attribute the origin of the unicorn to India.

Italy: Etruscan goddess mounted on a bull. Bronze. Roman Museum.

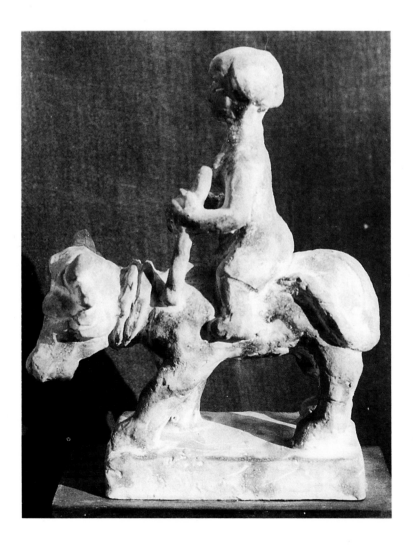

The Animal and Plant Forms of the God

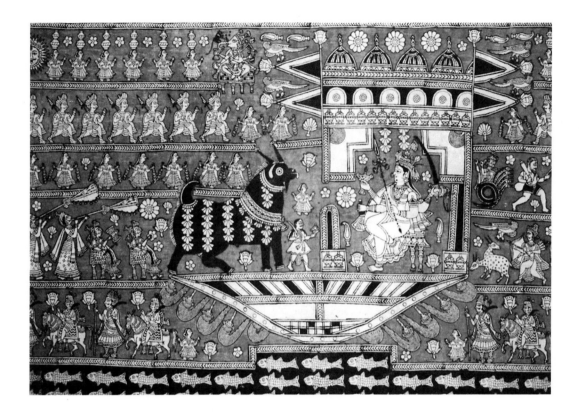

India: The great goddess venerates the lingam and welcomes Shiva and the bull. Printed fabric, nineteenth century. Madras. Collection of Jacques Cloarec.

"We worship he who unites the weak and the strong, he who disturbs and is never disturbed, the bull Nandi with his large hump and his resplendent single horn" (*Linga Purāna,* 1.21.25).

Humpbacked bulls associated with Shiva's lingam from the Chalcolithic period have been discovered by A. Stein in Gedrosia (the Quetta region in contemporary Pakistan). In a similar vein, images of an ithyphallic Shiva standing on a bull's horns have been found in the Kazbek treasure in the mountains of the Caucasus.

"In the land of the Canaanites, in Ugarit, the principle deities were the bulls El and Baal. Baal corresponds to the Phoenician Hadad, the Syrien-Hittite Théshub, and the Egyptian Seth. Baal goes into combat with monsters with a human body bearing the head of a bull" (R. F. Willetts, *Cretan Cults and Festivals,* p. 162). The El cult practiced by Hebrew patriarchs emigrated to Palestine, where it was proscribed by Moses but survived until the reign of David. Statues of sacred bulls, influenced by Egyptian art, go back to that era and reflect the survival of these ancient beliefs in the Semitic world. Testimony confirming the persistence of ecstatic dances is evident in the epoch of Samuel (1020 B.C.).

The cows Apis and Mnevis, living incarnations of the cult of Osiris, played a fundamental role in the religion of the Egyptians, who were themselves Semites, at least by language. According to Cicero, a second Dionysus was born of Hapi or of Serapis, a Nile god in bull form. The pharaoh was called "the bull who makes the mother fruitful."

In Elide, Dionysus-bull was invoked. He was viewed as appearing from the sea in the guise of a dancing bull. According to the Shaivite myth, it is Nandi, the bull, who teaches dance and music to men. As Athena noted in *Deiphosophistes* (11.5.476a), Dionysus is very often described by the poets as a bull, and though he is not only a god-bull, he willingly embodies himself as such. In Crete, as in Egypt, the cow was the symbol of the Moon, and the bull, the Sun—the one who impregnates. In Olympus, Dionysus was worshiped under the form of a bull or a serpent. We can see representations on Greek vases of Dionysus and Poseidon mounted on two bulls, one white and the other black. "Parallel and analogous to such symbolisms may be the imagery common to cattle-herding peoples of the bull or goat as the male principle of fertility distributing his sexual favours and energy among female devotees and initiates. The early western Asiatic cult of Dionysus is one example, and another is the cult of the Celtic horned god Cernunnos" (Philip Rawson, *Primitive Erotic Art*, p. 54).

There are also folk legends concerning the birth of the bull. In the *Kanda Purānam* (6.13.303), in the Tamil tongue, the goddess of fortune, Lakshmī, feared drowning after a flood. This fear prompted her to adopt the form of a bull, which would become the mount of Shiva.

Shiva is always represented either mounted on or accompanied by a bull. The bull that wanders in search of adventure personifies the force of the erotic. Shiva, who dominates the erotic, is the only one who can ride the bull. To obtain favors from the god, a bull is traditionally liberated. In India the entire bovine species is sacred. In Phrygia, as elsewhere in ancient times, it was a criminal offense to kill a bovine animal. The cow and the ox were sacred. Bull festivals, bull cults, and bull sacrifices are everywhere remnants of Shaivite rites and the phallus cult.

In Minoan Crete, the bull games were part of a cult. The sacred bull-fights were praised in songs heard on the terraces of the palace. The paintings of Knossos show acrobats stunt-riding bulls. The bull personified honesty and justice—the virtues of the powerful. Nandi symbolizes dharma, the cosmic order. The same role is attributed to the

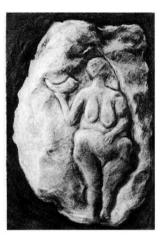

primordial buffalo by the Sioux. In the Hellenistic world, infants were dedicated to bulls. Spartan children of different ages ate and slept together, forming a community called a herd *(agela)* under the surveillance of a young man called the head bull *(bouagoi)*. During the festival of Thiodaisias, which was associated with the passage of young men from their *agela* and their collective marriage (according to Strabo), the god worshiped was the Minoan god-bull, later called the Cretan Zeus (Kretagenus). In the thiases, Dionysian associations such as that of Torre Nova (A.D. 200), roles of *boukolos* (herdsman) and *archiboukolos* are manifestations of a return to the Dionysian bull cult. The divine bull was finally sacrificed, as was the Minotaur by Theseus—the god put to death for the redemption of men. Its blood was then carefully gathered into a chalice.

The bull is the manifestation of Dionysus in the animal kingdom. The god incarnates within the most masculine and noblest of all animals, by virtue of which, when placed on the altar of sacrifice, he brings redemption to the world.

In Shaivite India, the sacrifice of the bull is rarely practiced today, but it is an essential part of the ancient ritual. In Rome, the sacred character of the bull and the sacrificial rites were perpetuated in Mithraicism until about A.D. 500. The Spanish bullfights, with their bull killings, are a survival of the Mithraicism that was very widespread in the Roman armies.

HORNS

As the bull's symbolic representation, the horn represents power, strength, and virility. We find its representations in the very depths of prehistory. From Laussel (ancient Perigord, circa 27,000 B.C.), at the height of the Ice Age, an image of a goddess holding a bull's horn has been discovered (Marshack, *The Roots of Civilization*, p. 335). The Egyptian *Book of the Dead* calls the god Amon the "lord of the two horns." In Hebrew, *queren* means "horn," "potency," and "strength" at the same time. In the Psalms, the horn signifies the power of God, the strongest defense of those who invoke it (Psalms 18:14).

In Chinese myth one comes across the terrible Tch'e Yeou of the horned head. In Mohenjo Daro the ithyphallic god appears in a yoga posture wearing bull horns. In Ugarit, on a stela predating Christ by fifteen centuries, the god called Misericordia, the potent Bull, is repre-

ABOVE
France: Goddess holding bull's horn, circa 27,000 B.C.
Illustration by Jim Ann Howard.
OPPOSITE
Crete: Head of bull, 1450 B.C.
Photograph by Leonard von Watt.

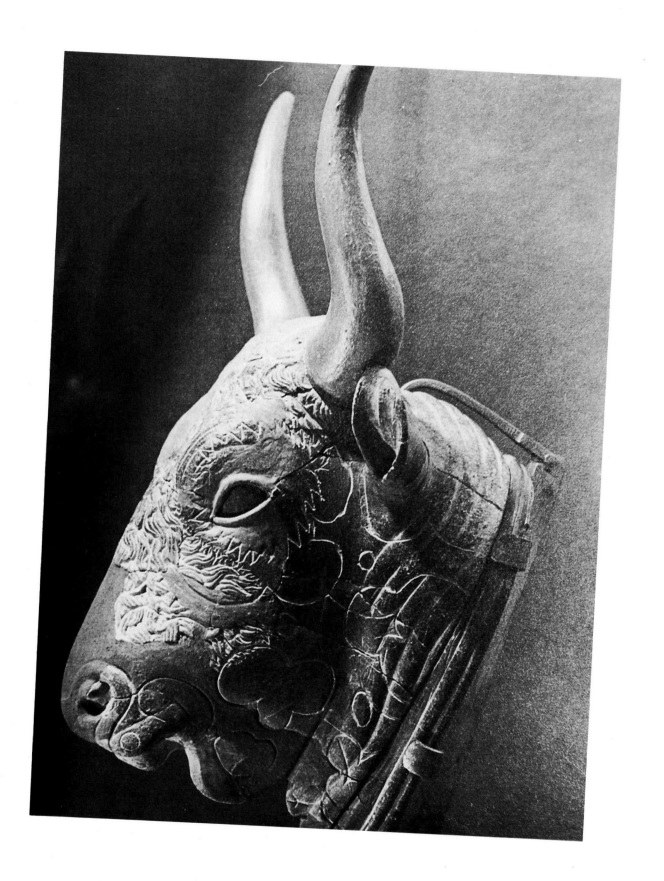

sented seated upon a throne. The portraits of kings were ornamented with horns to show that they took their powers from heaven. The Cretan royal family had a bull-god as its ancestor. The bull became the symbol of royalty; that is why we find the portraits of kings surmounted by horns.

The Macedonian kings bore horns as a mark of their divine origin. When Moses descended from the mountaintop filled with the spirit of God, his head appeared to be adorned with horns. (Exodus 34:35). The cloister of Vaison-la-Romaine has a carved head of Christ wearing two large horns. In the Babylonian epoch, Gilgamesh went to war against Khumbalba, a giant whose head was adorned with horns. The ox Apis in Egypt was the representation of the god-king. Reshap, the warrior god of Asian origin identical with Seth, the brother of Osiris, bears the crown of Upper Egypt decorated with two horns. According to Cauvin, ritual bull skulls found at Mureybed, in the Mid-Euphrates region, date from 8200 B.C. In Russia and Bulgaria there are horns of consecration that date from about 3890 B.C.

Dionysus is represented as a horned god: "Zeus . . . spared him a shelter in which he could be born. He concealed him within his thigh, fastening him in with golden buckles. . . . When the time fixed by fate arrived, the father brought forth the bullhorned god and crowned him in a coil of serpents" (Euripides, *The Bacchae*, 95–102).

The royal Etruscan ossuaries carry horns in the guise of decorations on the rooflines. In Delos there exists, in addition to the cubical stone, an altar called the Keraton, which was made from the horns of cattle and goats and was consecrated to the cult of Apollo Karneios, the protector of horned animals. In Brittany this cult reemerges as that dedicated to St. Corneille, worshiped in the Carnac region. "The very name of *corne* (horn) is manifestly linked to the root KRN and to *couronne* (crown), another symbolic expression of the same idea. . . . Both are "peaks" and are placed on the head. . . . Similarly, the Greek word *keraunos,* lightning, which normally strikes the summits, high places, and elevated objects, seems a derivative of the same root" (René Guénon, *Symboles fondamentaux de la science sacrée*, p. 204). The name Carnac, a center of megalithic temples, is also evocative of the KRN root, as are the Egyptian Karnak and the Indian Konarak.

Warriors of various countries, notably the Gauls, have worn horned helmets. Alexander is represented as Amon with horns that symbolize the divine nature of his genius.

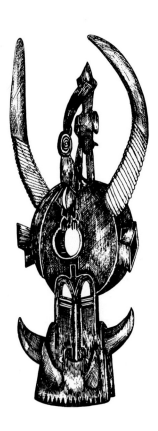

Africa: Ritual horned mask with phallic figure. Senufo.

The significance of horns extended throughout the pre-Celtic, Celtic, and Germanic world as far as central Germany. "Kernunnos, or Cornely, patron of horned beasts, is the builder of the megalithic monuments next to which are found the *mein gurun,* 'lightning stones,' as prehistoric axes are commonly referred to by the local inhabitants. The cult of Saint Cornely, sacrificed for his faith, evokes the image of the Minoan sacred bull and his attributes—the horns and the double-bladed axe" (Gwenc'hland Le Scouezec, *Guide de la Bretagne mystérieuse,* p. 170).

The horned demon of popular folklore, with his cloven hooves and brandishing a trident, is without a doubt of the same origin. Horns as a symbol of divine might are encountered in Africa as well.

THE LUNAR CRESCENT

Shiva's bull horns are represented by the crescent moon that he bears on his forehead. A Cambodian inscription designates the moon as the perfect horn of Shiva's bull. This assimilation is also to be found in Sumer, in Babylon, and in Egypt. For the Hindus, as for the Semitic peoples, the moon is a male deity. The moon god of Ur was called "the Mighty Young Bull of Heaven" or "the Mighty Young Bull with Robust Horns." Sin, the lunar god of Mesopotamia, took the form of a bull. In Egypt the divinity of the moon is called "The Bull of the Stars." Osiris, the lunar god, was represented by a bull. Equally, the moon is the cup that holds the nectar of immortality *(amrita)* and the terminal point of the ancestral path *(pitriyāna).*

In Persia, the moon was called *Gaoeithra,* the cup where the primal bull deposited his semen.

THE HEALER GOD AND THE SERPENT

A serpent surrounds the lingam and, with its forked tongue, touches its orifice. Shiva wears a necklace of serpents. The snake is the image of the slumbering, latent energy, the source of sexual and mental prowess, which is found curled up at the base of the spine, utilized by the yogi in the course of his interior voyaging to aid him in his attempt at conquering the upper worlds. Serpents protect Shiva; he wears them as ornaments and as his sacred belt. According to the

The Animal and Plant Forms of the God

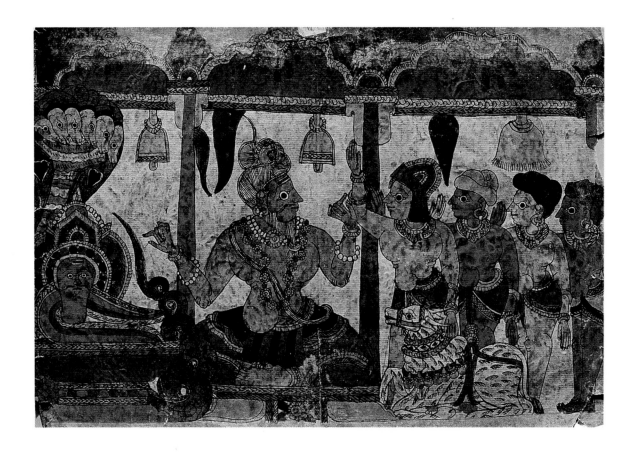

India: Painting of linga worship, nineteenth century. Photograph by Lance Dane.

Griya Sūtra, a collection of texts concerning household rituals, offerings to Shiva should be made in those areas frequented by snakes. Only Shiva, the healer, can control them. The serpent distills poison, which is the counterpart of *amrita,* the elixir of immortality, a poison that prevents the human being from achieving liberation.

Rudra-Shiva, god of the plant world, knows every remedy. He is depicted as the greatest of doctors (*Rig Veda,* 1.45.4; 1.114.5; 2.33.2, 4, 7, 12, 13, etc.). He prepares poisons but has no fear of them himself. When the gods and titans gave birth to the world by their churning of the cosmic ocean, Shiva drew out the poison as well as the nectar. The poison remained stuck in his throat, which as a result turned blue. That is why Shiva is also called the blue-throated god *(nīla-kantha).* The healer effects his cures through the prudent use of poisons. The snake, being the bearer of the most virulent poisons, thus becomes the necklace of Shiva, who has an eternal association with serpents. This aspect of the god is to be found in Rome in Asclepios. "The cult of Asclepios was already important in Crete. The serpent is his companion. The respect for Asclepios and for his miraculous, medical cures ... was so enduring that in the last pagan era he was considered Christ's principal adversary" (R. F. Willetts, *Cretan Cults and Festivals*, p. 224).

The snakes are inhabitants of the world underground. They live in the entrails of the earth and know its secrets. They are the possessors of poison and consequently are the antithesis of the celestial deities who possess ambrosia, the elixir of eternal life. The ancient Dravidians worshiped the serpents who made up the great Naga people, represented everywhere with a human body and a serpent's tail. These images are very numerous on the temples, and they play a large part in Shaivite legends. At times snakes will mix in human affairs. In the *Nāgananda*, "The Happiness of the Serpent," the poet Harsha recounts the adventures of a young Naga rescued from Vishnu's cruel vulture by a heroic prince, thanks to timely intervention by the goddess.

It is the Naga who preserve the prestigious sciences of ancient sages and the secrets of magical powers. The *Shatapatha Brāhmana* (13.4.3, 9) (circa 1000 B.C.) recognizes that the true wisdom, "the Veda, is in fact the knowledge of serpents." Snakes are survivals of the most ancient gods.

The serpent, or Naga, cult was incorporated into the Aryan religion during the period of the sūtras (600–400 B.C.). "When Alexander attacked and conquered various Indian cities, he discovered in certain ones, besides other animals, a snake that the Indians considered sacred. They guarded it in an underground site and worshiped it devotedly. They begged Alexander not to let anyone disturb it, and he consented" (Aelian, *Variae Historiae*, chap. 21).

"The serpent cult is associated . . . with that of underground powers, sometimes fertilizing and benevolent, sometimes dreadful, because, according to their whim, they insured or destroyed the stability of the world" (Paolo Santarcangelli, *Il libro dei Labirinti*, p. 112). A serpent is entwined with Hermes' wand. Two snakes encircle Mercury's caduceus and Esculape's healing wand. Asclepios is accompanied by a serpent, which serves as an indication of his magic power and a reminder that the healing sciences were originally the province of ancient god-snakes.

Uraus, the snake that the Egyptian rulers carried in the guise of a diadem, symbolized the healing power associated with royalty. The sovereigns of Asura bear an identical diadem in the iconography of Hindu temples.

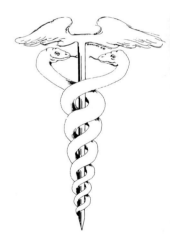

Caduceus. Illustration by Oswald Simmonds, Jr, from Sule Greg Wilson's The Drummer's Path *(Destiny Books).*

The Animal and Plant Forms of the God

"Certain Dionysian congregations have retained and renewed the tradition of familiarity with reptiles and snake handling, a practice whose ancestry and religious nature is attested to in the Aegean world by monuments dating from the Minoan second millennium" (H. Jeanmaire, *Dionysos,* p. 403). "Snake charmers" have always been numerous in India, where they are not merely a tourist attraction but form a brotherhood to which magical powers are attributed.

The serpent cult can be found even today in Italy. In Abruzzi, for the festival of Saint Dominic, snakes are wrapped around the saint's statue. In a custom that is obviously inherited from a more ancient ritual, the faithful manipulate the serpents while following the statue in a procession.

The most important of the Minoan household cults was that of the serpent, particularly in the form of the serpent goddess, the mistress of animals. The old serpent goddess cropped up beside Zeus in the form of Hera. The snake became a male deity in the Greece of a later era but remained at the center of the household cult. The Cretan Zeus in serpent form is called Meilikhios, the Benevolent. As an image of the female principle, the snake represents attachment to the things of the earth. "In all traditions, the snake is the master of women because it is the symbol of fecundity" (Mircea Eliade, *Histoire*).

In the Greek myth related by Athenagoras (20.292), Zeus is in pursuit of his mother, Rhea. Since she has taken the form of a snake, he does too, and uniting with her in what has come to be called the "knot of Hercules," he takes possession of her. In western Asia, Astarte is represented as having snakes entwined around her hands and arms. In India, Kali appears covered in snakes.

Among the Tchokwé peoples in Angola, a wooden serpent is deposited on the nuptial bed. Among the Nourouma of Gangora, a woman is believed to become pregnant if a snake enters her hut. In India, women wishing to conceive adopt a cobra.

THE LINGAM-SHARIRA, OR SEXUAL CODE

In Yoga, "the subtle center situated at the base of the spine is a triangle of desire, knowledge, and action, which forms the womb at whose heart rises the phallus that is born of its own self, shining like a thousand suns" *(Shiva Purāna).*

The living individual is but a transitory moment of the permanent

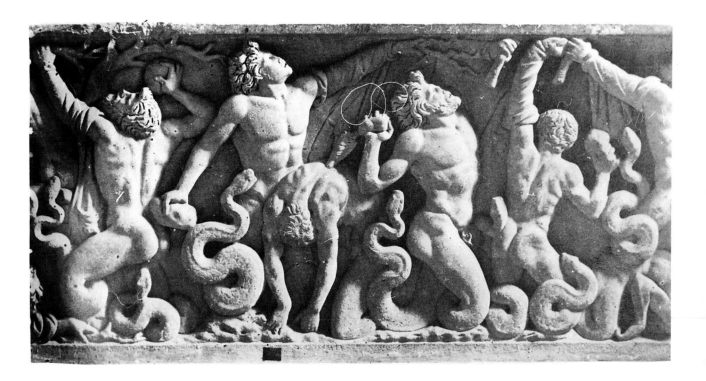

reality that is the species. Individually insignificant, each living being is essential as a link in the chain. He is like the bearer in a relay of the Olympic torch. He is the conveyer of a permanent model and code that is transmitted from one individual to the next. The chief characteristic of life is the aptitude to reproduce: to continue and to transmit. It evolves across thousands of generations. Man is called *linga-dhara,* the phallus bearer. He is the sex organ's servant. His individuality is of no importance save in the very limited capacity in which he adds several new elements to the code he has received and must send on within the framework of the species to which he belongs. He may be only a link in the chain, but there are good links that reinforce the chain and bad links that weaken it. The permanent transmissible element, the code that defines the possibilities of each individual, each link, is part of the semen that he transmits. It is issued from man's sex just as the universe is issued from the lingam, the divine phallus. According to the renowned treatise of Shaivite cosmology, the *Sāmkhya-Kārikā,* "the program, the sexual body exists before the physical development of its bearer. It contains the seed of the intellect and other faculties as well as physical characteristics. But it can embody them only when it becomes incarnate, even though it remains independent of the body. It is characterized by a *dharma,* a "goal to

Italy: Bas-relief depicting myth of The Iliad. *Rome. Vatican Museum.*

The Animal and Plant Forms of the God

achieve," which is transported with it when it is transmitted from one body to another. In order to achieve this goal assigned to it in the creation, the sexual code, the *lingam-sharira,* incarnated by the power of nature *(pradhāna),* acts like an actor who plays one role after another" (*Sāmkhya-Kārikā,* 41–42).

"The universe results from the relations of a phallus and a womb, of a form and a substance. Everything, consequently, carries the signature of the lingam and the yoni. It is the deity who, under the form of individual phalluses, penetrates all wombs and procreates every being" ("Lingopāsanā Rahasya").

The principle called Shiva represents the totality of all procreative power to be found in the universe. "It is he alone that penetrates every womb" (*Shvetāshvatara Upanishad,* 5.2).

It is in the sperm that all the physical and mental characteristics of the individual are summarized. Therefore, what the Hindu call the phallic body is what we call DNA.

According to Galen, whose opinion was prevalent during the Middle Ages, the semen originates in the brain, descends the length of the spinal cord, and leaves by means of the phallus, the center of the body and the source of life.

◆

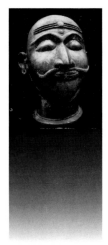

8

NAMES AND ASPECTS OF THE ITHYPHALLIC GOD

In the forest the name of the tiger is never pronounced; by the same reasoning the name of a god is never overtly stated. He is evoked only indirectly by adjectives. The word *dieu* (god) itself comes from the root *div*, meaning "radiant."

"In the *Aitareya Brāhmana* (ii, chapter 34, 7), it is prescribed that a formula must be altered from the form in which it occurs in the *Rigveda* in order to avoid the direct mention of the name 'Rudra' of the god. In another passage of the same text, it is interesting to note he is never named, but is referred to as 'the god here', and the same avoidance of the direct use of the name is also to be seen elsewhere" (P. Banerjee, *Early Indian Religions*, p. 49). That is why, in every mythology, the god-phallus is invoked under multiple names.

In the Indian pantheon, Rudra, "the Howler," refers to his terrible aspect, and Shiva, "the Protector," to his favorable one. Following the aspect of the faithful's preferred god establishes the secret and magical formula to be communicated to the apprentice at his initiation—a formula that will be his constant companion and recourse all the rest of his life.

Dionysus also appeared under his multiple aspects as a bull god, a god having a double birth, a horned god, and sometimes as a young Dionysus riding a panther.

Shiva, the ithyphallic god, is Prathamajā (first-born), the "eldest of the gods," and is also called Bhāskara (luminous), corresponding to the Phanos (he who illuminates) of the Orphic tradition. He engendered Skanda (the jet of sperm), the god of beauty and of the mysteries, also called Murugan or Kumāra (the adolescent), the equivalent of the Cretan Kouros (lad). He is Guha (the mysterious) whom the Greeks called Hermes.

THE ANDROGYNOUS GOD (ARDHANARĪSHVARA)

In the process of creation, "the power of conception *(vimarsha)* and the power of realization *(prakāsha)*, when united, are embodied first in a point limit *(bindu)*, a localization that is the departure point for time-space. From here is issued the vibration or sound *(nāda)* which is the substance of the universe. Space is a female principle, a receptacle; time is an active male principle. Their unity, symbolized by the divine hermaphrodite, represents Eros (Kāma), the creative impulse" (Karpātrī, "Shrī Shiva Tattva").

Primordial divinity is essentially bisexual. The division of the principle into two polar opposites is merely an appearance. The divine is defined in the Upanishads as "this in which the opposites coexist." "When Shiva and Shakti are united, their unity is sensual pleasure. Sensual pleasure is their reality; their existence apart is only fiction" (Karpātrī, "Lingopāsanā Rahasya").

The reality of the world is therefore essentially sensual pleasure, the spark produced by the union of opposites. The hermaphrodite, image of the nondivision of opposites, represents absolute, pure, and permanent sensual pleasure, which is divine nature. "Bisexuality is one of the multiple formulas of totality-unity signified by the union of opposing pairs: masculine-feminine, visible-invisible, heaven-earth, light-darkness, but also goodness-wickedness, creation-destruction, etc." (Mircea Eliade, *Histoire des croyances et des idées religieuses,* p. 178).

"The first creation consisted of spirits, genies, and demons issued from the mouth of the uncreated being as a materialization of his vital breath *(prāna)*. Rudra appeared first, as luminous as the rising sun. He was androgynous.... The Immensity, on seeing this divine hermaphrodite, said to it: 'Divide yourself.' It was thereby with the god's left side

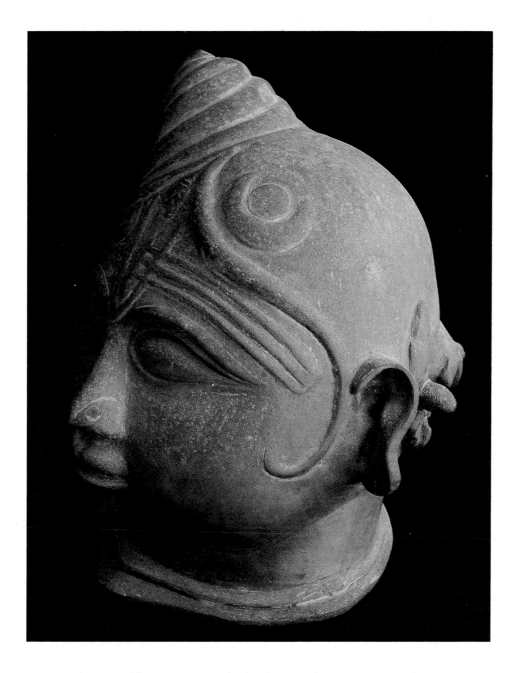

that a goddess was created who became his companion" (*Linga Purāna,* 41.41−42 and 99.15−19).

In order to procreate a world outside of itself, the deity divided itself in half, and the two poles drew away from each other. The state of absolute happiness disappeared and is recreated only by the union of opposites, by love. The divine hermaphrodite "divided its body into two halves, one male, the other female; the male in that female procreated the universe" (*Manu Smriti,* 1.32).

India: Bronze Shiva linga sheath, late eighteenth century. Photograph by Lance Dane.

Names and Aspects of the Ithyphallic God

89

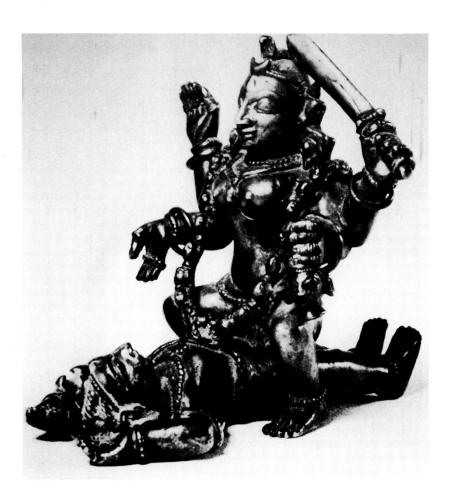

India: Brass statue of Shiva and Shakti, circa eighteenth century. Photograph from Rufus Camphausen's Encyclopedia of Erotic Wisdom *(Inner Traditions).*

The initial principle can be conceived of as either masculine or feminine, as a god or as a goddess, but in either case it concerns an androgynous or transsexual being.

According to the Phrygian tradition related by Pausanias (7.17.10–12), Papas (Zeus) fertilized a stone phallus named Agdos, and the latter engendered a hermaphroditic being named Agditis. The gods, by castrating Agditis, transformed it into the goddess Cybele. She is the equivalent of Pārvatī, the lady of the mountains, the feminine counterpart of Shiva. Among the Canaanites at Ugarit, Anat, like other goddesses of love and war, is provided with masculine attributes and is considered bisexual. This is also the case with the Etruscan goddess. The Hurrite god Kumarbi is bisexual, like the Akkadian gods Tiamat and Zarvan. The Hittite Teshub, son of the celestial god Anu, is an androgynous deity. Images of hermaphroditic and ithyphallic deities from the Neolithic era are encountered everywhere. A wooden sculpture found in Somerset, England, is a typical example.

All degrees of bisexuality appear in the aspects of the god, virile in his terrible form, effeminate in his joyous and benevolent aspects. On the other hand, the goddess can appear virile and aggressive like Bhairavī or Kālī, the destructive power. In this case she plays the active role in her relations with Shiva, with whom she practices *viparīta maithuna,* inverted copulation. Again, by contrast, the goddess is modest, feminine and sweet when she appears as the lady of the mountains (Pārvatī) or Satī (Fidelity).

The same applies to Dionysus, who is sometimes represented as a bearded man in his prime, sometimes an effeminate adolescent. "At the opportune moment, Zeus undid the stitches on his thigh and gave birth to Dionysus, whom he entrusted to Hermes and had sent to Ino and Athanas, telling them to raise him as a girl" (Apollodorus, *Bibliothèque,* 3.4.3). Dionysus is captured by a barbarian king, who mocks him for his feminine appearance. According to Nicander, it was under the guise of a young girl that Dionysus warned the Minyades, who were absurdly hard-working and virtuous, not to neglect his initiation rites.

In a text of Aeschylus (fragment 61) the king cries out on seeing him: 'From where do you come, man-woman, and what is your country? What is this you're wearing?' The clothing that symbolized his double nature was removed: the saffron-colored-veil, the belt, the gold miter. He was stripped naked, though not stripped of his virility, but he was too fragile to give it value."

Hercules, the most virile of heroes, exchanged clothes with Omphalos. Arjuna, the valorous prince of the *Mahābhārata,* during his exile, disguised himself as a eunuch and taught music and dance to the daughter of King Virata.

In the myth cited by Aristophanes and retold by Plato in the *Symposium,* the first men were androgynes. As punishment for their rebellion, Zeus divided them in two. In the same vein, according to the Purānas, the first men were sages, who were still kindred of the deities and who engendered their sons by a kind of mental projection. It was to destroy their power, which the celestial beings believed threatened their own, that the gods created woman and reproduction by sexual union. In Genesis, the creation of the woman from one of Adam's ribs implies the androgynous nature of the original man, created in the image of the divine hermaphrodite.

Like Shiva, the first man, Adam, was man on his right side and woman on his left. All the Tantric rituals in which women participate are called left-handed rituals. The left side is man's weak side and is reserved for humble or impure tasks. That is why one never extends the left hand to be shaken. To offer an object with the left hand is viewed as a sign of derision. The circumambulation of a god's image must be done keeping to its right side—in other words, clockwise. In Tantric magic, when the feminine aspect of the divinity is to be invoked, this is done in the reverse direction. Every bisexual being can be considered an emanation of the transcendental aspect of the god. The androgyne, the homosexual, the pervert had a symbolic value and were considered in ancient civilizations to be privileged beings, images of the Ardhanārīshvara. Under this title they played a special role in magic and Tantric rituals, as in shamanism. "The final goal of Tantrism is the reunion of the two polar principles, Shiva and Shakti, in one's own body.... Initiatic androgeny is not always signified by a physical operation, as is the case among the Australians. In many cases it is suggested by the dressing up of boys as girls and girls as boys.... The homosexual practices attested to in various initiations are probably to be explained by a similar belief, the knowledge that the neophytes, during their initiatic instruction, combine both sexes" (Mircea Eliade, *Mephistophélès et l'Androgyne*, pp. 139 and 149).

Among shamans, divinatory power is linked to bisexuality. In the ritual gesture of the *anasyrma*, the magician dressed as a woman lifts up his robes to expose his sex, thus appearing as an androgyne. The Etruscan prophet carried a phallus attached to her belt. In the mysteries of Hercules Victor, in Italy, the god as well as the initiates were clothed as women. Cross-dressing was supposed to promote health, youth, and vigor and to lengthen life expectancy.

"In Siberian shamanism, the shaman symbolically combines the two sexes.... The shaman conducts himself as a woman, dressing in female clothes and at times even taking a husband. This ritual bisexuality—or asexuality—is supposed to be simultaneously a sign of spirituality, of commerce with the gods and spirits, and a source of sacred strength.... The shaman symbolically restores the unity of heaven and earth, and consequently maintains the communication between gods and men. This bisexuality is lived ritually and ecstatically; it is assumed as an indispensable condition for surpassing the condition of the profane man.... Siberian and Indonesian shamans reverse their sexual comportment in order to live *in concreto* ritual androgyny" (Eliade, *Mephistophélès*, pp. 144–45).

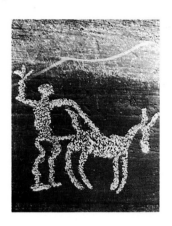

Italy: Rock carving from a sacred site at Val Comonica. Photograph by Mission E. Anati from Philip Rawson's Primitive Erotic Art *(Weidenfeld & Nicolson).*

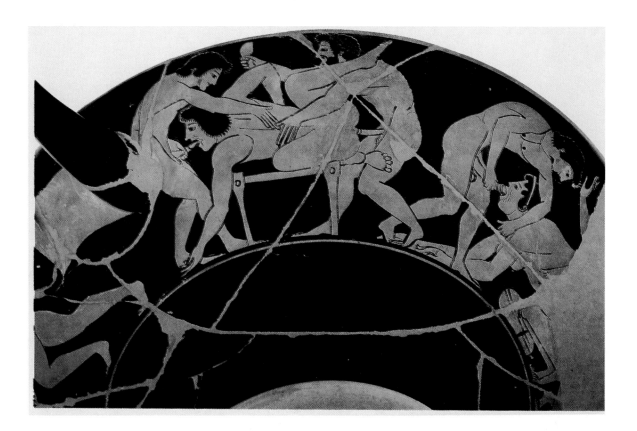

Greece: Attic cup, late sixth century B.C. *British Museum.*

"One cannot become a sexually adult male without having experienced the coexistence of the two sexes, androgyny; in other words, one cannot attain a way of particular and well-determined being without having experienced a way of total being" (Eliade, *Mephistophélès,* p. 138).

The goal toward which the human species should aim is the progressive reintegration of the sexes until androgyny is obtained. The evolved being tends toward bisexuality. In the bisexual being, the communication between the two halves of the brain is particularly well developed. That is why the creative artist is often a bisexual, as are the mage and the medium, whence the role of those called "inverts" in magic rites and the importance attached to the rituals "of the left hand" in Tantric practices.

The myth of the divine androgyne is symbolically represented by the phoenix, which engenders itself and therefore represents immortality. When Christianity implanted itself in Rome, the phoenix became associated with the image of Christ. When the universe is reabsorbed, the two opposing principles will again be one; the hermaphrodite will reconstitute itself, first in the creatures and then in the divinity itself.

Names and Aspects of the Ithyphallic God

93

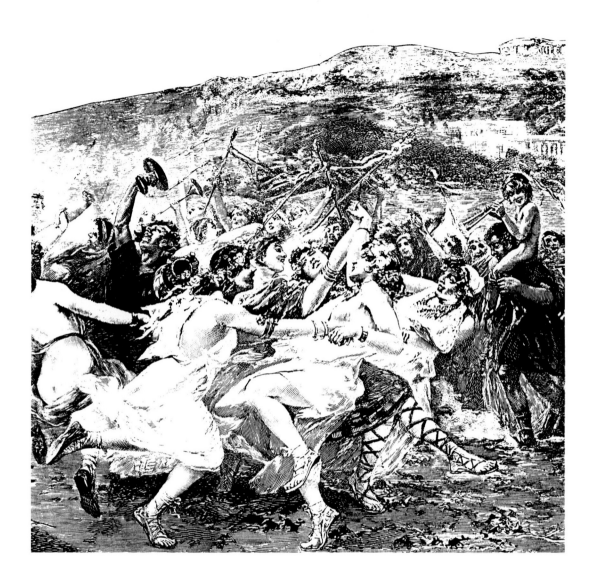

*Bacchanalia festival.
Illustration by Jim Harter.*

Among the Dogon and the Bambara of Mali, the hymen is the materialization of man's female soul. An analogous belief is probably the
origin of the practice of circumcision among the Semites.

THE PHALLOPHORIAS, FESTIVALS OF SPRING

Phallic processions and the installation of votive phalluses in Greece
were part of the festivals of Dionysus, god of the suppression of bans
and taboos. During the sixth century, Heraclitus of Ephesus remarked
that if the procession and the phallic songs had not been in honor of
Dionysus, they would have been embarrassing. Herodotus, who in

Egypt had witnessed processions escorting the image of a phallic deity, concluded that the cult of Dionysus had come to Greece from Egypt. The rural Dionysiac festivals basically consisted of the promenading of a large-scale wooden phallus. The retinue was formed of figures wearing animal masks. Obscene jokes accompanied these spectacles. Aristophanes, in *The Acharnians*, gives a humorous version:

Diceopolis has concluded a personal arrangement that has allowed him to demobilize and return to the joys of civilian life. With his daughter as a canephore (basket-bearer) and his slave Xanthias as a phallophore (phallus-bearer), he gets ready to celebrate his own personal Dionysiac festival, which the war has too long deferred. He puts his little retinue in order, then begins intoning a canticle in which the phallus is personified under the name of Phales:

"Gather round, gather round . . . you, the canephore a couple of steps farther ahead. You, Xanthas, hold that phallus straight up. Put the basket down, my dear, so we can make the sacrifice. . . .

"My master Dionysus, accept with favor this procession and this offering, which I and my family, released from war's misery, now hold to celebrate the Country Dionysias. May it bring blessing upon us, and may this thirty-year truce I have concluded bring me naught but happiness! Ah, daughter, carry the basket gracefully . . . and with proper solemnity! Ah, a happy lad is he who will someday kiss you and make you fart, like a weasel, when you wake. . . . Now get going, and watch out in this crowd that no one sneaks up on you and lifts your jewels. Xanthias, it is up to both of you, the phallus and yourself, to stay perfectly upright, behind the basket-bearer. And me—I am singing the chant of the phallus. You, wife, watch from the terrace! Keep moving! Phales, comrade of Bacchus and his dinner companion, nightcrawler, adulterer, lover of boys, it has been six years since I've invoked you in my village with my songs. It is because I've made my personal truce with the Spartans and sent all my troubles packing to the devil. I won't be troubled any more by the war and the 'let's go to war.' Ah, now may things get better, Phales, Phales, as when one has caught the pretty slave girl from next door stealing some wood, then catches her in the rocks, grabs her around the waist, lifts her up and gives it to her! Phales, Phales, if after my party you need another drink to get your feet back under you, tomorrow morning, we will have a good potful and my shield will be hung peacefully over the hearth."

In the Dionysian comedies of fifth-century Athens, the phallus, proudly displayed by the actors and satyrs of the retinue, was one of the trumps for success. The satyrs played flutes and displayed improbable erections.

At the time of village-organized phallophorias, several phalluses were promenaded. On a vase displayed at the Florence Museum, an enormous phallus can be seen, fixed on a sort of altar carried on the shoulders of ithyphallic figures. Participants climb on the phallus, which is made of a wooden beam whose end is carved in a gland-like form with an eye painted on its side. Ropes allow the phallus to be maneuvered and twitched about. An important phallophoria, one to which foreigners were invited, took place at the time of the Grand Dionysia of Athens; it is likely that the idol was better sculpted and more richly adorned.

Athena, according to Callixenos of Rhodes, described a procession that took place in Alexandria, under the rule of Ptolemy II Philadelphia with an incredible splendor, that assembled together hundreds of participants and paraded more than ten sacred chariots before the luxurious pavilion that had been erected for the occasion by order of the king. An army of Sileni, satyrs, "ithyphalli," and maenads accompanied the god's images. Tableaus celebrated his prowess or exalted the gifts that he brought to mankind. In an Indian triumphal march of Bacchus, strange beasts and men of faraway lands were paraded. According to the narrator, "on another chariot was a golden thyrsus ninety cubits long and a silver lance of sixty cubits" and on another chariot was "a golden phallus one hundred twenty cubits long, covered with engravings and adorned with gilded strips, with a gold sun, six cubits in circumference, at its tip." The festival of Floralia took place in Rome at the beginning of May.

The spring festival is the festival of Shiva. The festivals of Shiva are always the festivals of the humble and low-born. At the time of Holi, the spring festival that corresponded to Dionysia and of which carnivals are a survival, craftsmen and servants had the right to insult and mistreat their patrons, the nobility and the priesthood. This was done with the aid of many curses and obscenities. The Gana, Shiva's youngsters, did likewise with regard to the gods, sages, and brahmans. At the time of these festivals, large red painted phalluses and images of ithyphallic apes were paraded about. A figure dressed in white, representing Shiva, led the retinue mounted on a donkey. The participants flooded the

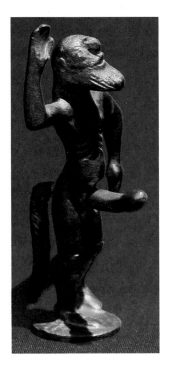

Thailand: Bronze ithyphallic ape.

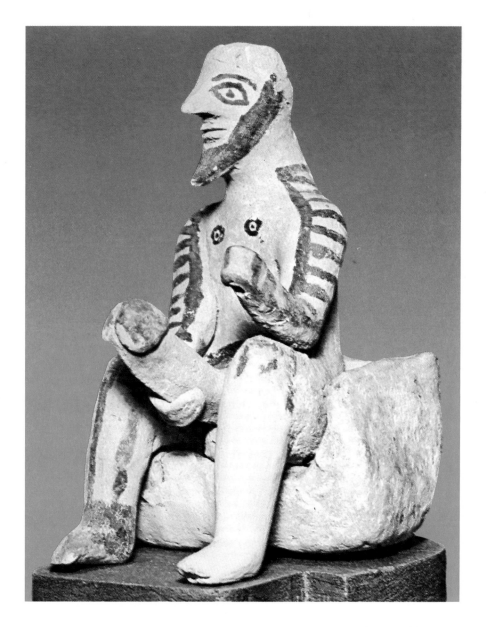

spectators with jets of colored water, which brings to mind the confetti used at carnivals in the West.

In Rome, for the festival of Liberalia, the phallus Liber was transported across the countryside and the city on a chariot. Obscene remarks were a prelude to the erection of a phallus in the Lavinium forum. Saint Augustine mentions that in the course of the Liberalia an enormous phallus was paraded on a magnificent chariot covered with garlands of flowers. At the time of the Lupercalia, in honor of Faunus and Priapus, the naked Luperchs made the circuit of the Pelation, whipping the women with lashes to make them fecund. The festivals

Greece. Clay satyr. National Archeological Museum, Athens.

Names and Aspects of the Ithyphallic God

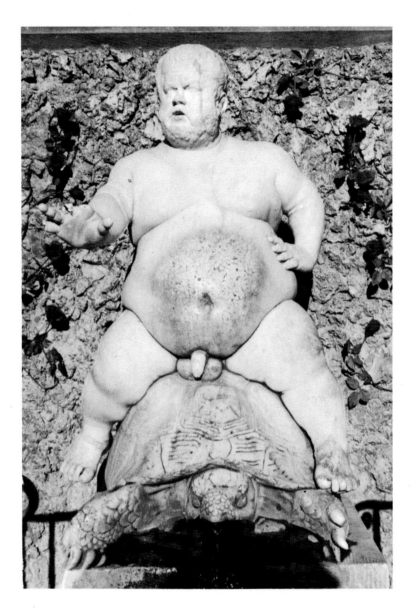

Italy: Statue of an obese nude, identified with Bacchus. Pitti Palace, Florence.

in honor of Bacchus and Osiris were called phallic. The Bacchanalia took place in Rome at the time of the grape harvest, October 23 to 29. The phallophores were the ministers of Bacchus who bore the phallus at the time of his festivals.

THE UNIVERSAL NATURE OF THE CULT

The phallus cult, which seems to have spread throughout the entire world during prehistoric times, has long perpetuated itself, even into the present, in various regions of the world.

Phallic representations in Egypt, Greece, and Italy are countless. The monumental sculptures of Delos are among the most famous. Images of the phallus are to be found wherever the Roman Empire established itself. Nimes remained for a long time the center of the Priapus cult in southern Gaul.

In Sweden, the principal seat of the cult was in Uppsala. Adam de Brème, in his eleventh-century work *De Situ Daniae,* wrote that "the third of the Uppsala gods was Fricco, who was represented by a large phallus and spread peace and pleasure among mortals." On the occasion of a marriage a sacrifice was offered to Fricco.

Phallic images are to be found everywhere throughout Southeast Asia as well as in Indonesia and the entire Melanesian and Oceanic

Indonesia: Ithyphallic wood statuette. Collection of Jacques Cloarec.

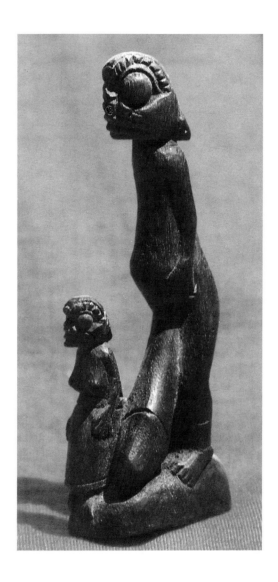

Names and Aspects of the Ithyphallic God

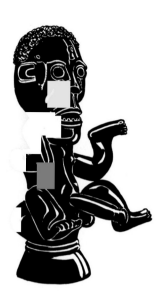

Nigeria: Headdress crown used as a mask. Repoussé leather.

world. Phallic images can be encountered in the isles of Oceania, including Easter Island.

In Melanesia the phallus is worshiped in Sepik and in Borneo. Ithyphallic stone figures are still worshiped in New Guinea,whence a gold phallus comes as well. Phallus-shaped fish hooks are used by fishermen to catch sharks. The Polynesian statues of Hawaii, the Cook Islands, and the Tonga Islands are similar to those of New Guinea.

In the Americas, ithyphallic Mayan deities can be discovered in Mexico and Arizona. Stone phalluses were worshiped in Costa Rica and in Jamaica, where birds with male sex organs were also worshiped. An image of an ithyphallic dancer, dating from the beginning of this century, has been found in Colima, Mexico. Others of a more recent provenance come from the Taino. In Panama the Cuno Indians wear ritual bark costumes with large penises. From Peru comes a mortar in the form of a snake with a pestle in the form of a phallus. The vast numbers of erotic pottery pieces in Mexico, however, do not seem to be of a religious nature.

"Among Siberian peoples (e.g. the Kumandin) a horse-sacrifice is accompanied by a performance by masked men wearing huge wooden phalli" (Philip Rawson, *Primitive Erotic Art*, p. 19).

More recently, in Cambodia, in a ceremony called the Popil ritual, the faithful circumnavigate a plateau, representing a vulva, crowned with a candle, representing the phallus. In Japan little stone phalluses are buried to ensure prosperity. In China it is a piece of triangular jade, the *kwei*, which is equivalent to the Hindu lingam.

Phallic altars are found in the majority of African countries. "In Ethiopia the phallic symbolism has perpetuated itself in the steep valleys that descend toward northern Kenya, where numerous monoliths are found that have been sculpted to resemble the phallus. Certain of them go back to the Bronze Age and are contemporaries of the ones at Stonehenge or Carnac, but others are relatively modern. Phallic tombstones can be found in the Bagiuni Islands off the coast of Somalia, but they are more likely to be found farther to the south, in particular at Bagamoyo and Tanganyika.

"The fact that many of the minarets of the mosques on the northern part of the coast are indubitably phallus-shaped adds an indigenous flavor to the East African culture, which remains, however, typically Islamic" (Basil Davidson, *Old Africa Rediscovered*, p. 184).

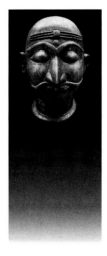

9

◆

THE SURVIVALS

"Antiquity made Priapus into a god; the Middle Ages made him into a saint, who, under several names, remains present throughout the Christian world. In the Midi of France and in Provence, Languedoc, and the Lyonnais region, Priapus continues to be worshiped under the name of Saint Foutin, to whom the Priapian attribute was transmitted under the form of a large wooden phallus. The cult of this saint, as it was practiced in the seventh century, is described by Pierre de L'Estoile in *La Confession de Sancy* (fifth volume of Henry III's Journal). We learn there that phalluses dedicated to Saint Foutin were suspended from the chapel ceilings. When the wind agitated them they produced a soft murmuring, which at times disturbed the serenity of devoted souls.

"In Embrun, in the High Alps, women poured libations of wine on the head of Saint Foutin's phallus. When the wine collected there turned to vinegar it was then employed for a use that is only obscurely alluded to. When the Protestants took Embrun in 1585, they found the phallus preserved among the relics of the church, the head still reddened from the ablutions of wine. Another phallus, covered with hide, was the object of a cult in the church of Saint Eutrope in Orange. The

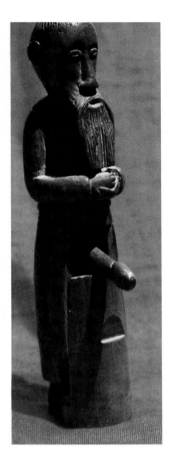

ABOVE
France: Folk art of clergyman
with member. Wood with secret
compartment. Collection of
Jacques Cloarec.
OPPOSITE
France: Folk art of monk
inserted inside a phallus.
Terracotta.

Protestants seized it and burned it publicly in 1562" (Payne Knight, *The Worship of Priapus*, p. 66).

"Near Clermont, in Auvergne, an isolated rock can be found that has the shape of a large phallus and is called Saint Foutin. Analogous phallic saints were worshiped under the names of Saint Guerlichon or Greluchon, in the diocese of Bourges, Saint Gilles in the Cotentin, Saint Remy in Anjou, Saint Regnaud in Burgundy, Saint Arnaud and especially Saint Guignole near Brest, and in the village of La Chatelette in Bercy.

"Very many of these phalluses were still an object of worship in the eighteenth century. Certain among them were worn down by the continual rubbings employed upon them to obtain their powder" (Payne Knight, in *The Worship of Generative Power*, p. 133).

In Antwerp, Belgium, until relatively recently, Priapus was worshiped under the name of Ters (a word of unknown origin but identical in meaning with the Greek phallus or the Latin *fascinum*). Joannis Goropius, in his *Origines Antwerpianae* on the antiquities of Antwerp, in the middle of the sixteenth century, explains why the Ters was worshiped by the people of Antwerp: "When women drop an object, fall down, or if some unexpected accident frustrates them, even the most respectable invoke Priapus with loud cries under his obscene name to obtain his protection. On the door of the city prison can be found a statue that had been provided with a phallus that is now entirely worn away" (Joannis Goropi Becani, *Origines Antwerpiae* [1569], 1.26–101).

Abraham Golnitz, in his *Itinerarium Belgico-Gallicum* (1631) mentions a phallus at the entrance to the cloister of the church of Saint Walpurgis in Antwerp, which had been constructed on the site of an ancient temple dedicated to Priapus. The Antwerp citizens, at certain times of the year, decorated this phallus with flowers and came to scratch it to obtain the powder, which was used as a remedy against sterility.

In Montreux, near Carpentras, in a twelfth or thirteenth century church is a phallus of Saint Didier that is celebrated on the second Sunday in May. Moreover, in the same region and still worshiped even today is Saint Gens, within a grotto shaped like a vagina. Young men take the image of the saint and race with it several kilometers to the grotto. There they take water and mix it with their sperm, which they then try to induce the woman of their choice to drink. The emblem of Saint Gens is a plowshare pulled by a wolf and a cow.

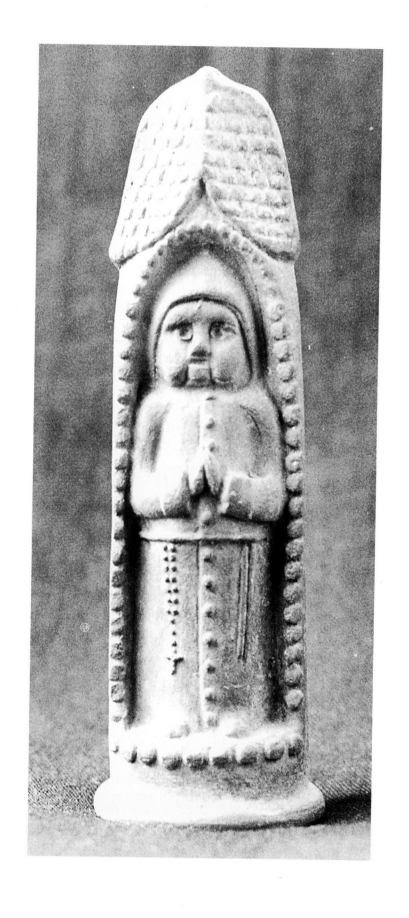

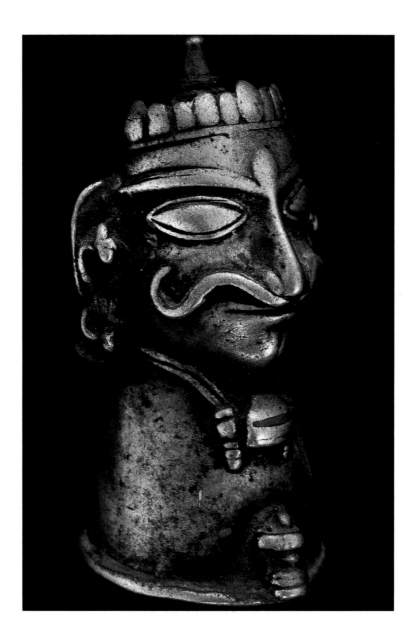

India: Shiva personified
on his linga. Bronze, late
eighteenth century. Photograph
by Lance Dane.

According to Daulaire, until relatively recently, in the village of Saintes on Palm Sunday, which was called the Festival of Penises, phallus-shaped biscuits were distributed.

Sir William Hamilton, an English resident of the Naples court, in a letter dated December 30, 1871, recounts that in Isernia, near Naples, for the festival of Saints Cosmas and Damien on September 27, a phallus that was prudishly called Saint Cosmas's big toe was displayed in the church. Wax phalluses were sold as good luck charms.

The rites of Priapus, used to combat livestock disease, continued in England until the thirteenth century.

"At the beginning of 1882, between March 29 and April 5, a priest of the parish of Inverkeithing, Scotland, celebrated the rites of Priapus by gathering the young women of the town together and making them dance around the god's statue. Parading a wooden image of the male organ of generation, he himself sang and danced while accompanying his song with gestures and attitudes adapted to the surrounding circumstances, and encouraged licentious acts from the participants with words that were no less so. The more timid of those in attendance, scandalized by these proceedings, reproached him, to which he responded in derision. Cited to appear before his archbishop, he excused himself, explaining that it was local custom, and he was granted leave to keep his post" (*Chronicle of Lancercosted*, p. 109).

The custom of carrying small phalluses as protection against bad luck and pernicious influences, widespread among the Romans, persisted throughout the Middle Ages and has never been completely abandoned. It has been a constant practice among the Gypsies. In Italy the phallus is sometimes replaced with a horn. In France, in a note on the decorated lead figures found in the Seine and collected by Arthur Forgeais (Paris, 1858) we learn that "almost all these phalluses have wings; one of them has bird feet and claws, and another has a sort of bell hanging at its neck. These objects are analogous to Roman phallic ornaments discovered in Pompeii. One is a representation of a woman astride a horse on top of a phallus with human legs; another has dog legs. One of them represents a little man with an enormous phallus.

"In San Agatha di Gaeti, near Naples, a gold-handled cross has been found composed of four phalluses. It has been constructed to be suspended and must have belonged to some powerful individual. In Italy these phallic amulets are in common use and are sold daily, in Naples, for one carlo each, which is the equivalent of four pence in English money or four French centimes. One of them, as can be seen, is entwined by a serpent. They are considered so effective in safeguarding the personal security of those who carry them that perhaps there isn't a Neapolitan peasant who doesn't make a habit of carrying one in his coat pocket.

"There is yet another less evident emblem of the phallus, which has ruled as an amulet since time immemorial. Antique dealers have called it the phallic hand. The ancients had two forms of this hand, one in which the middle finger was extended while the thumb and other fingers were folded back, and the other in the form of a fist but with the

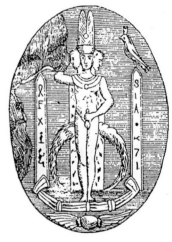

The god Osiris taking the phallic oath. British Museum. Illustration from Rufus Camphausen's Encyclopedia of Erotic Wisdom *(Inner Traditions).*

The Survivals

thumb passing between the index and middle fingers. The first of these forms is the more ancient. The extension of the finger represents the extension of the *membrum virile,* and the fingers folded back on either side represent the testicles; this is why the Romans called the middle finger the *digitus impudicus* or *infamis.* To display one's hand in this form was considered the most contemptuous of insults, because it designated the person to whom it was addressed as one given to vices that went against nature. This was also the significance attributed to it by the Romans" (Payne Knight, in *The Worship of Generative Power*).

The Roman carnival inherited Priapus, whom it transformed into Pulcinella (Punch) of the stiff-bearded chin and pointed ears. The Italian ethnologist Annabella Rossi has published a study on the phallic and hermaphroditic character of Pulcinella, whose name comes from *pollice* (thumb). Like Attis and Mithra, he in fact wears the *pileus,* the pointed cap that is characteristic of the phallic cult mysteries. He is called *cetrulo* (cucumber) in reference to the vegetable of phallic significance. He also holds a horn. His humpback, which brings good luck, is considered a sign of hermaphroditism.

"In Martano, in Lecce province, on Easter Sunday, people seeking a cure go to a chapel where a menhir is to be found and have to pass through a hole in the stone. Such healing, by sliding through a hole or through a narrow space between two stones, is a prehistoric rite that is to be found throughout the whole of Europe" (Alphonso di Nola, *L'Arco di Rovo,* p. 44). Currently in southern Italy the locals introduce the word *cazzo,* like an invocation, into the most common phrases: "Che cazzo vuoi" (what do you want).

PHALLUS WORSHIP

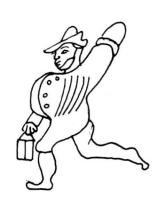

One century after the birth of Jesus, Plutarch reported that a mysterious voice, heard by a sailor, announced the death of the great god Pan. This news froze the Greco-Roman world with horror. The phallic god, the father of all the gods, risked dragging the civilized world with him in his fall, leaving men without protection. A new era opened up, full of dangers and conflicts, which little by little would lead to the extinction of the human race.

The phallus cult, born of the great religion that from Neolithic and Bronze Age times had spread from India to the farthest borders of Europe, remained anchored secretly in man's soul. Despite its persecu-

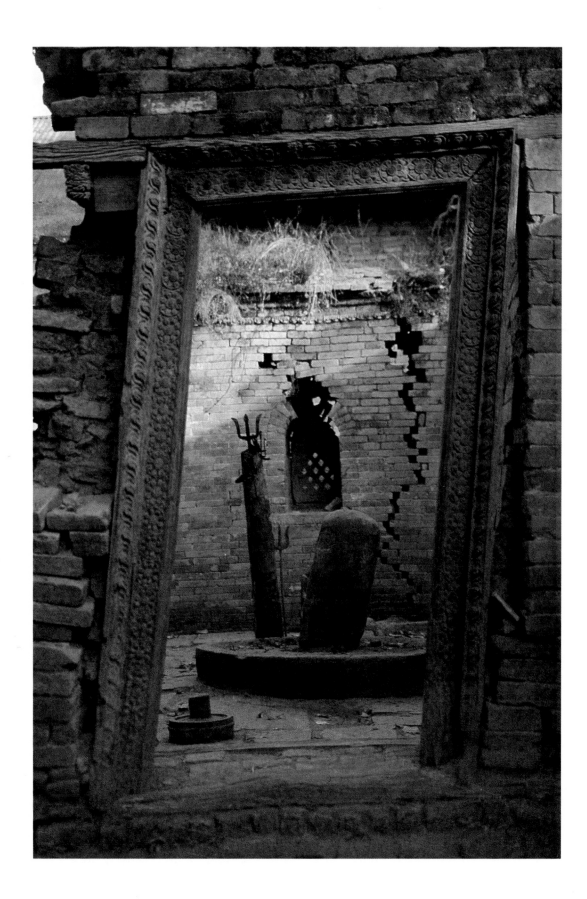

tion, we rediscover the cult of the divine phallus in rites, festivals, ceremonies, survivals, vestiges, and the traces it has left in its path, sometimes disguised but nevertheless always present.

Just as the eye, organ of vision, has the form of the sun, and the ear, organ of sound perception, has the form of the labyrinth, the form of the phallus, tree of life, whose sap gives birth to living beings, is the most fundamental of symbols. The form of the phallus corresponds to that of the Universe. It represents the visible prolongation of the unknowable being whom, according to the *Purusha Sūkta,* "it surpasses in size by ten fingers" *(atyatishtati dasangulam).*

All ancient peoples endeavored to comprehend and analyze the characteristics of the organs whose union gave birth to living beings, and they reproduced the mystery by which the creator gave birth to the world.

Only he who worships the lingam, the upraised phallus within the vulva, respects the creative principle and, by means of this symbol, is capable of attaining divine reality.

"The lingam is an external sign, a symbol. However, it must be considered that the lingam is of two kinds: external and internal. The cruder organ is the exterior, while the subtle organ is the interior one. Simple folk worship the external lingam and concern themselves with its rituals and sacrifices. The goal of the image of the phallus is to waken the faithful to knowledge. The immaterial lingam is not perceptible to those who see only the surface of things. The subtle and eternal lingam is perceptible only to those who have attained knowledge" (*Linga Purāna,* 1.75.19–22.) "Those who practice the ritual sacrifices and faithfully worship the physical lingam are not capable of controlling their mental activity by meditating upon its subtle aspect. . . . Those who have not yet gained awareness of the mental sex organ, the subtle sex organ, must worship the physical sex organ, and not the reverse" (*Shiva Purāna, Rudra Samhitā,* 1.12.51–42).

By domination of the sexual instinct, we can acquire physical and mental prowess. Through sexual union, new beings can come into existence. This union represents a link between two worlds, a bridge where life is embodied and where the divine spirit is incarnated. The form of the organs that accomplish this ritual is the most important of symbols. They are the visible form of the creator. "By worshiping the lingam, one is not deifying a physical organ; one simply recognizes an eternal and divine form manifested within the microcosm. The human phallus is the image of the causal form present in all things. Those who

THE PHALLUS

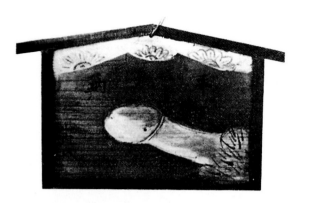

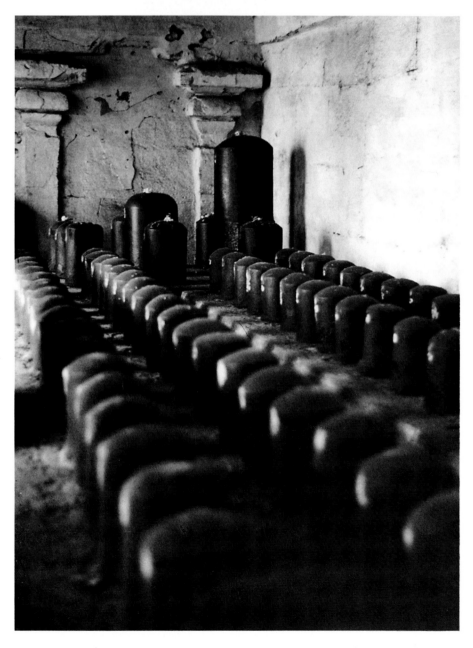

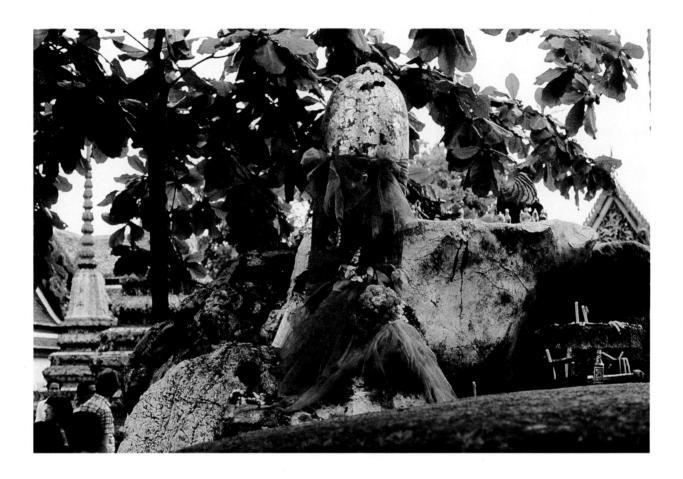

Thailand: Shiva lingam near Buddhist shrine, garlanded with colored silks, flowers, and other offerings. Photograph by Nik Douglas.

wish not to recognize the divine nature of the phallus, who understand nothing of the importance of the sexual rite, who consider the acts of love as vile and contemptible or as a simple physical function, are certain to fail in their attempts at spiritual or material realization. To ignore the sacred character of the phallus is dangerous whereas by worshiping it one obtains pleasure *(bhukti)* and liberation *(mukti)*" ("Lingopāsanā Rahaysa").

"He who lets his life pass by without having honored the phallus is in truth a pitiable, guilty and damned being. If one were to weigh on a scale, with one side holding the adoration of the phallus and the other holding charity, youth, pilgrimages, sacrifices, and virtue, it would be the adoration of the phallus, source of pleasure and liberation, as well as a sure protection against adversity, that would outweigh the other side" (*Shiva Purāna,* 1.21, 23—24, and 26).

"He who worships the phallus knowing that it is the primal cause, the source of consciousness and the substance of the Universe, is closer to me than any other being" *(Shiva Purāna).*

The cult of the phallus is recommended in the *Mahābhārata*: "From whom comes the semen offered in sacrifice at the birth of the world in the mouth of Fire, the mouth of Agni, teacher of the gods and the anti-gods? Is the gold mountain Sumeru created from another semen? Who other than the ithyphallic god wanders naked throughout the world? Who else can sublimate his procreative power? Who else has made his beloved half of his self and cannot be vanquished by Eros? It is Rudra, the god of gods who creates and destroys. Can you thus see, O king of heaven, why the entire world carries the signature of the lingam and the yoni? You know as well that the changing worlds are issued from the sperm of the lingam during the act of love. All the gods, genies, and powerful demons whose desires are never slaked recognize that nothing exists outside of that-which-gives-bliss (Shankara) . . . the sovereign of the worlds, the cause of causes. We have never heard that the phallus of anyone else was adored by the gods. Who is therefore more desired than he whose phallus is worshiped by Brahmā, Vishnu, and all the gods, as well as yourself?" (*Mahābhārata; Anushāsana Parvan*, 14.211–232).

For the rites of lingam worship, the faithful brought fresh flowers, pure water, shoots of herbs, greenery, and sun-dried rice. They attached particular importance to the purity of the cult objects and to the physical cleanliness of the worshiper.

Why is the lingam worshiped? Because it is a symbol of permanence, an archetypical image that reveals the nature of the universal man, Purusha. To worship the phallus is to recognize the presence of the divine in the human. It is the opposite of an anthropomorphic monotheism, which is the projection of human individualism onto the divine. In the instrument of procreation we worship the creative principle, and we do this joyfully because this organ is also the instrument of a pleasure that for a fleeting instant gives us a glimpse of divine beatitude. The divine state is composed of three elements: existence, consciousness, and sensual pleasure *(sat-chit-ānanda)*. Only sensual pleasure forms part of the domain of immediate experience. Therefore, by its intermediation we are able to sense, we are able to touch, the divine state.

The phallus cult implies the worship of harmony, the beauty of the world, the respect of the divine work, and the infinite variety of forms and of beings in which the divine dream is embodied. It reminds us that each of us is but an ephemeral being of little importance, that our sole role is to improve the chain that we momentarily represent in the evolution of the species and to pass it on. The cult of the phallus is therefore linked to the recognition of the permanence of the species in regard to the transitory nature of the individual, to the principle that establishes the laws whence we are issued and not their accidental and temporary applications. It is awareness of the life principle as opposed to the living individual, and of the abstract over the concrete. The worship of the phallus has implications on every level, whether of morality, ritual, cosmology, or society. Renouncing phallus worship in favor of a person, whether divine or human, is a form of idolatry, an outrage toward the creative principle. All the sacred texts of Shaivism, the Purānas, the Tantras, and the Agama tell us over and over again that only those who faithfully practice phallus worship will be saved, that

India: Temple at Sangameshvara, early seventh century. Photograph by Lance Dane.

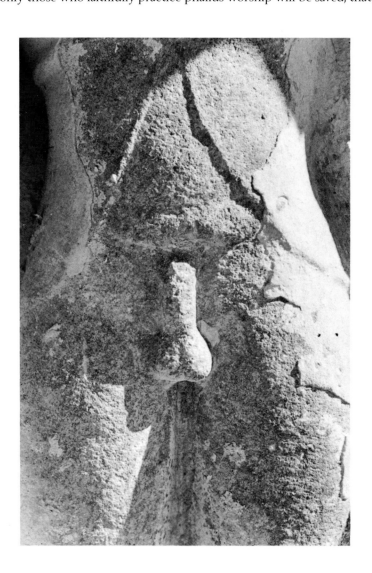

all societies that draw away from the phallus cult and respect for physical sexuality are destined for decline and will be annihilated like the Asura, the race of men that preceded contemporary humanity.

For the man possessed by the love of nature and the quest of the divine who successfully liberates himself from the taboos, superstitions, prohibitions, and myths of modern religion, the phallus—image of the creative principle—will appear anew as a luminous and eternal symbol that is the source of joy and prosperity.

Leonardo da Vinci noted, on several occasions, the respect that is owed to the virile member: "Man is wrong to be ashamed of mentioning and displaying it, always covering and hiding it. He should, on the contrary, decorate and display it with the proper gravity as if it were an envoy."

After a life of failures and setbacks on the religious, moral, material, and social planes, Maurice Sachs wrote:

"I hope to know no other temple than nature, to adore naught but the sun, to worship only the radiant member that creates man" (*Le Sabbat*, p. 177).

The Alexander of Michel Tournier's *Les Météores* (p. 105) proclaims:

"I cannot imagine God as anything other than a hard penis raised high, seated on the base of its two testicles as a monument erected to virility, the creative principle, the Holy Trinity, an idol of horn hanging at the exact center of the human body. . . . trifoliate flower that is the emblem of the passionate life, I will never be done singing your praises."

◆

GLOSSARY OF SANSKRIT TERMS

Ākāsha Space or ether; region of pure consciousness.

Alingam Without marks.

Amrita Nectar of immortality.

Ānanda Sensual pleasure; transcendent bliss; spiritual ecstasy.

Ardhanārīshvara Androgynous.

Argha Vagina.

Avyakta Nonmanifestation.

Bāna Arrow.

Bhāskara Luminous.

Bhukti Pleasure.

Bīja Seed; semen; primary cause.

Bindu Point limit, where all living beings unite.

Chandra Moon.

Chit Consciousness.

Dharma Cosmic order.

Guha Mysterious.

Hinkāra Invocation of the god.

Kāma Eros.

Kirti Glory.

Kumāra Adolescent.

Lāngala Spade.

Linga-dhara Phallus-bearer.

Lingam, linga Phallus.

Mahā Transcendent.

Mahat Universal consciousness, the "great principle."

Maithuna Copulation; union of Shiva and Shakti.

Mukha Face.

Mukti Liberation.

Nāda Vibration, sound.

Nandi Joyous; the bull.

Nidhana Closing hymn.

Nirālamba Independent divinity.

Nirvikāra Beyond change.

Pāsha The bond, the snare.

Pashu Livestock.

Pati Master.

Pitriyāna Ancestral destiny.

Prakāsha Power of realization or expression.

Prakriti Nature; creative energy; female principle.

Prāna Breath.

Prastāva Vedic hymn of praise.
Prathamajā First born.
Pratihāra Chorus.
Purusha Cosmic man.

Sailaja Standing stone.
Sāmkhya Cosmology.
Sat Existence.
Satī Fidelity.
Shālagrāma Pebbles with a
  phallic significance.
Shankara That which gives
  bliss.
Shisna-deva God-phallus.
Shūdra Artisan caste.
Skanda Jet of sperm.

Soma Elixir, ambrosia.
Sthānu Column.

Udgītha Vedic hymn of glory.
Upastha Penis.
Urdhva-linga He of the erect
  penis.

Vimarsha Power of conception.
Viparīta Inverted position for
  copulation.
Vīrya Virile essence.

Yajña Kunda, hearth.
Yoni Womb.

BIBLIOGRAPHY

SANSKRIT TEXTS

Yajur Veda.
Taittirīya Samhitā.
Purusha Sukta.
Chhāndogya Upanishad.
Shvetashvatara Upanishad.
Taittirīya Upanishad.
Bhāgavata Purāna.
Linga Purāna.
Shiva Purāna.
Skanda Purāna.
Bhagavad Gītā.
Mahābhārata.
Nārada Pancharātra.
Manu Smriti.
Sāmkhya Kārikā.
Harsha (theater), trans. A. Daniélou.

TAMIL TEXTS

Kanda Puranam.

HINDU TEXTS

Kavirāj, Gopinātha. "Linga Rahasya." *Kalyana,* Shiva Anka, 1937.
Karpātrī, Svāmī. "Lingopāsanā Rahasya"; "Shrī Shiva Tattva."
    Siddhānta, Benares, 1939.

HEBREW AND BIBLICAL TEXTS

Genesis, Leviticus, Numbers, II Samuel, Joshua, Jeremiah, Sephir Bahir, Sephir Yezirah.

CLASSICAL TEXTS

Aelian, *Variae Historiae*.
Aeschylus, *Fragments*.
Athenagoras, *Legatio pro Christianis*.
Apollodorus, *Bibliothèque*.
Aristophanes, *The Acharnians*.
The Epic of Gilgamesh.
Euripides, *The Bacchae*.
Hesiod, *Works and Days*.
Hesiod, *Theogony*.
Pausanias, *Periegis*.
Plato, *The Banquet*.
Sophocles, *Ajax*.

ENGLISH TEXTS

Anonymous. *The Worship of Generative Power*. London, 1825.
Banerjee, P. *Early Indian Religions*. Delhi, 1973.
Davidson, Basil. *Old Africa Rediscovered*.
Graves, Robert. *Greek Myths*. London, 1958.
Marshack, Alexander. *The Roots of Civilization*. London, 1976.
Knight, Richard Payne. *The Worship of Priapus*. London, 1786.
Rawson, Philip. *Primitive Erotic Art*. London, 1973.
Willets, R. F. *Cretan Cults and Festivals*. New York, 1962.

ITALIAN TEXTS

Boardman, John, and Eugenio La Rocca. *Eros en Grecia*. Mondadori; French version: Laffont, 1976.
Colli, Giorgio. *La Sapienza Greca*. Milan, 1977.
Nola, Alfonso di. *L'Arco di Rovo*. Turin, 1983.
Rossi, Annabella. *Carnevale si chiama Vicenzo*. Rome, 1977.
Santarcangeli, Paolo. *Il libro dei Labirinti*. Florence, 1967.

FRENCH TEXTS

Chevalier, Jean, and Alain Gheerbrant. *Dictionnaire des symboles*. Paris, 1982.

Daniélou, Alain. *Le polythéisme hindou.* Paris, 1975.

Daniélou, Alain. *Shiva et Dionysos.* Paris, 1979.

Daniélou, Alain. *La Fantaisie des Dieux et l'Aventure Humaine.* Paris, 1985.

Dulaure, J.-A. *Des Divinités génératrices ches les Anciens et les Modernes.* Paris, 1825; reprint: Pardès, 1985.

Dupuis, Jacques. *Au Nom du Père.* Paris, 1987.

Eliade, Mircea. *Histoire des croyances et des idées religieuses.* Geneva, 1976.

Eliade, Mircea. *Mephistophélès et l'Androgyne.* Paris, 1962.

Evola, Julius. *Le Yoga tantrique.* Paris, 1971.

Guénon, René. *Symboles fondamentaux de la science sacrée.* Paris, 1962.

Jafkar, Amin. *Saint Gens, enfant de Monteux.* Paris, 1984.

Jeanmaire, H. *Dionysos.* Paris, 1951.

Lambert, Jean-Clarence. *Labrynthes et dédales du monde.*

Le Scouezec, Gwenc'hland. *Guide de la Bretagne mystérieuse.* Paris, 1966.

Mercadé, Jean. *Eros Kalos. Grèce,* Paris, 1976.

Scholem, G. C. *Les Origines de la Kabbale;* trans. Jean Loewenson, Paris, 1966.

Vieyra, Maurice. *Les Religions de l'Anatolie antique.* Paris, 1953.

GERMAN TEXTS

Karlhans, Frank. *Der Phallus.* Frankfurt, 1989.

About the Author

ALAIN DANIÉLOU (1907−94), born in Paris, was the West's foremost interpreter of Hinduism. His father was a government minister and a friend of Aristide Briand; his mother was the founder of several schools of religious instruction; his brother became a cardinal.

Daniélou became involved with the artistic and musical milieu of Paris in the thirties, during which time he became close to Maurice Sachs, Henri Saguet, Jean Cocteau, and Pierre Gaxotte. After having been a painter, he studied dance with Legat, song with Panzera, and composition with Max d'Olonne.

Following a journey to Afghanistan he met Rabindranath Tagore and became fascinated by India, establishing residence in Benares in 1937. He resided there for more than fifteen years; converted to Hinduism; studied Hindi, Sanskrit, religion, and philosophy; and became an accomplished player of the vīnā.

On his return to Europe in 1958 he became an ardent champion of Eastern mystical music traditions and created the International Institute for Comparative Music Studies in Berlin and Venice to be responsible for the conservation and diffusion of these traditions. As Councillor of the International Council of Music he founded UNESCO's collection of traditional musics. In 1980 he retired to Italy, where he continued to write.

Daniélou is the author of more than thirty books about philosophy, religion, history, and the arts of India, including *The Complete Kāma Sūtra*; *Gods of Love and Ecstasy*; *Music and the Power of Sound*; *Myths and Gods of India*; *Virtue, Success, Pleasure, and Liberation*; and *While the Gods Play*.

◆